Special-Needs Kids Eat Right

Special-Needs Kids

Eat Right

Strategies to Help Kids on the Autism Spectrum Focus, Learn, and Thrive

Judy Converse
MPH, RD, LD

A PERIGEE BOOK

A PERIGEE BOOK
Published by the Penguin Group
Penguin Group (USA) Inc.
375 Hudson Street, New York, New York 10014, USA
Penguin Group (Canada), 90 Eglinton Avenue East, Suite 700, Toronto, Ontario M4P 2Y3,
Canada (a division of Pearson Penguin Canada Inc.) • Penguin Books Ltd., 80 Strand,
London WC2R 0RL, England • Penguin Group Ireland, 25 St. Stephen's Green, Dublin 2,
Ireland (a division of Penguin Books Ltd.) • Penguin Group (Australia), 250 Camberwell
Road, Camberwell, Victoria 3124, Australia (a division of Pearson Australia Group
Pty. Ltd.) • Penguin Books India Pvt. Ltd., 11 Community Centre, Panchsheel Park, New
Delhi—110 017, India • Penguin Group (NZ), 67 Apollo Drive, Rosedale, North Shore 0632,
New Zealand (a division of Pearson New Zealand Ltd.) • Penguin Books (South Africa) (Pty.)
Ltd., 24 Sturdee Avenue, Rosebank, Johannesburg 2196, South Africa • Penguin Books Ltd.,
Registered Offices: 80 Strand, London WC2R 0RL, England

While the author has made every effort to provide accurate telephone numbers and Internet
addresses at the time of publication, neither the publisher nor the author assumes any
responsibility for errors, or for changes that occur after publication. Further, the publisher does not
have any control over and does not assume any responsibility for author or third-party websites or
their content.

First edition: March 2009

Library of Congress Cataloging-in-Publication Data

Converse, Judy.
    Special-needs kids eat right : strategies to help kids on the autism spectrum focus,
learn, and thrive / Judy Converse.
        p.   cm.
    Includes index.
    ISBN 978-0-399-53488-1
    1. Autistic children—Nutrition—Popular works.   I. Title.
    RJ506.A9C6666 2009
    618.92'85882—dc22   2008041405

PRINTED IN THE UNITED STATES OF AMERICA

10   9   8   7   6   5   4   3   2   1

PUBLISHER'S NOTE: Neither the publisher nor the author is engaged in rendering professional
advice or services to the individual reader. The ideas, procedures, and suggestions contained in this
book are not intended as a substitute for consulting with your physician. All matters regarding your
health require medical supervision. Neither the author nor the publisher shall be liable or
responsible for any loss or damage allegedly arising from any information or suggestion in this book.

The recipes contained in this book are to be followed exactly as written. The publisher is not
responsible for your specific health or allergy needs that may require medical supervision. The
publisher is not responsible for any adverse reactions to the recipes contained in this book.

CONTENTS

3. Making Sense of Lab Tests | 66
Defining What to Do for the "One in Six"

4. Best of All Worlds Special Diet | 136
A Kid-Focused Way to Find the Right Diet Plan for Your Child

5. Supplements | 174
Medical Foods and Making Sense of a Dizzying Array of Options

6. Shop, Cook, Eat | 205
Making Nutrition Work in Your Kitchen

Introduction

A Nutritionist on the Front Lines

I'm a nutritionist. That's a fuzzy term that gets thrown around a lot by different health care providers of both strong and weak training and experience in it. What it means in my case is that I am a licensed registered dietitian with graduate and undergraduate degrees in nutrition from two universities. I completed 900 hours of supervised training in acute care settings (hospitals), outpatient clinics, and community public health programs such as WIC (the Supplemental Food Program for Women, Infants, and Children). It also means that per my registration and licensure boards, I must maintain 75 hours of approved continuing education hours every five years, or lose both credentials. No slacking off. I completed my graduate training in 1988, my registration status in 1989, and became licensed in 2001 (which was when my state began licensing nutrition professionals).

As fate would have it, I was also drawn into the Defeat Autism Now (DAN) community in 1998 and began provider training as soon as it was available. Soon after, I started something I never ever aspired to do, thought of doing, or wanted to do: I began a private practice, for children. This chose me more than I chose it. My own child, then two, had experienced struggles in infancy with feeding, illness, and developmental concerns that I had never heard of in all my training. I was astounded by how little attention our pediatric providers paid to the role of nutrition in his care, how uncurious they were about this piece, and how devoid of information they were about it. Even though I had already encountered many doctors in my training and my own health care who had not studied nutrition, it had never occurred to me that, of all disciplines, the pediatrician would be so disenfranchised from it. After all, if babies can't eat, or can't absorb their feedings normally, they can't sleep, grow, explore, learn, or develop typically. There is nothing more fundamental or essential to a baby's health than nutrition.

That was when my training really kicked into gear. I worked hard to right the challenges in my own house with infant and toddler feeding, allergy, growth, development, sleep, and behavior. This was in 1996. Not much of an Internet then. I lived in a coastal New England village with minimal library resources. Between cracking old texts and visiting the library at the Marine Biological Laboratory in Woods Hole, which either had or could order some of the scientific journals I needed, I began piecing answers together that worked well for my own child. As I did this, parents began approaching me for the same help. Of course, I wasn't the only mom in this boat. It simply floored me that, for families like mine, there was almost nowhere to turn for professional guidance on how nutrition matters for children. That is how Nutrition Care for Children came into being, a private practice I created to fill this gap.

It's still a tiny practice, but I am contacted now by families nationwide. The irony is that many parents tell me right up front that their child has no nutrition problems. Besides, they often add, the pediatrician has never mentioned any problem, and there are no bowel symptoms. I have never met a child with sensory processing disorder, autism, Asperger's, or ADHD with no nutrition problems, so I let parents discover with me what we can put right for their child, and then we watch the improvements unfurl. If they don't unfurl, then I hope they stay curious with me, and I make referrals to providers who can look at other layers. I would be the first person to tell a family there is no point to special nutrition measures for a child struggling with developmental, behavioral, growth, learning, or allergy problems. But so far, I haven't encountered a situation where nutrition care didn't help. We always find at least one lever worth pulling, one nutritional adjustment, and parents are glad to witness their child improve in ways large and small.

Whether your child has as grave a situation as autism, or a daunting but less challenging issue such as sensory processing disorder or nonverbal learning disability, nutrition tools can be effective allies. The nutrition care process is essentially the same for the whole gamut of behavioral, neurological, and developmental diagnoses the CDC says now affects one in six children in the United States today. Because we are talking about child nutrition assessment and care, and not psychosocial or educational evaluation tools, there is a reliable standard in place for this that has existed for decades. Blending this with what have become known as "biomedical" treatment tools makes for a powerful method of enhancing health and learning for these children, no matter what their developmental and learning diagnoses may be.

For parents of children with other special needs such as cystic fibrosis, diabetes, Crohn's disease, cerebral palsy, seizure disorders, or global developmental delay, this book might prove a useful read, too. Nutrition care for kids with these diagnoses is easier to access in today's medical landscape than it is for children with autism, so you may feel you have that base well covered. But there may be useful tidbits on the pages that follow—bits of information that might be overlooked by the staff at a major medical center, such as: Children with diabetes may show improvement in blood sugar control when using gluten-free diets; children with cystic fibrosis may have undetected inflammation from foods that further inhibits growth and gain; seizure disorders may improve with aggressive antifungal therapy or supplemental magnesium and pyridoxine. All children benefit from good nutrition support, but not all children get it. Most mainstream MD providers don't use it. All too often, it is not the focus of their training or a key aspect of their treatment methods.

Parents of children with autism face a bigger challenge in many ways, because the idea that nutrition supports apply to this condition is still bucked by many a doctor. Finding someone to work with your child on this can be difficult. If there is a silver lining to the autism epidemic, it may be that we are hearing the word "recovery" in the same breath as "autism." As hopeful as that is, many in the autism community bristle at it. While we talk about stroke recovery, cancer cure, diabetes cure, successful treatment for depression, or recovery from traumatic brain injuries, many stumble with "autism recovery," "cure autism," or even "autism is treatable." Some construe the very idea of recovery as a judgment on people with autism who don't want to change their unique talents or personalities.

To the contrary, my years in practice have convinced me that we should shed the view that autism is an inflexible, static affliction. It deserves the same determination for improvement that we fling at challenges such as diabetes, cancer, AIDS, or intractable depression. After years of watching children with autism spectrum or sensory challenges find joyful expression of their true personalities, or move toward higher functioning because of good nutrition care and biomedical tools, it is hard for me to remember that most MD providers and many parents are still out of this loop. Whatever your stance on this point, it works to focus on a goal everyone has: good health, contentment, and reaching one's potential, no matter what fate has thrown in your path. If a genetic predisposition has brought autism, cancer, stroke, diabetes, or Parkinson's disease into your life, or whether you view these conditions as entirely triggered by external factors, you are still here to live to the fullest and feel well. This is where therapeutic nutrition strategies really shine. Withholding these strategies from any child is illogical, and it's downright unethical if the child has signs and symptoms relating to nutrition or gastrointestinal (GI) problems.

As you will soon discover while you read this book, children with autism diagnoses, sensory integration disorder, or challenges with attention, focus, learning, mood, or behavior often have plenty of nutrition and GI problems. The science and practice that can repair or lessen nutrition and GI problems in children is not new, not novel, not fringy, and not alternative. The new part is looking at these children through this different lens. *Of course* children function better when problems found with this lens are fixed. Regardless of where you stand on the complex questions of why the diagnosis rates are exploding, or what causes autism, I hope we can agree that good nutrition is essential for all children—something we owe them and are capable of giving them, and something that can benefit them tremendously in their development and quality of life.

So, dive in. This book gives parents practical, straightforward information on approaching and using special diets for children with challenges such as autism, sensory integration disorder, attention problems, and more. The information here is based on everything I have been fortunate to absorb, experience, read, learn, and observe for over a decade in practice and as a parent. I am confident in the science that is already published on nutrition strategies for children with the kinds of problems now being found in autism spectrum disorders. For deeper reading on rationale, research, further biochemistry, or whatever you need to know more about, see the resources section, or visit www.NutritionCare.net for more information and support.

ONE

Engaging Your Providers

Working Together on Nutrition Care and Special Diets

Using nutrition therapies for a child with special needs can be complicated. Parents need support, guidance, expertise, resources, and encouragement for it, while providers need information they can work with to help you. It is a potent therapeutic tool that can work very well, or not work at all. Now is a good moment for pediatric providers of all stripes to learn about it. Thankfully, we already have highly applicable, well-pedigreed knowledge on child nutrition, plus constantly emerging new information about nutrition and autism, that we can put to use right now. But first, we have to close the gap between providers and parents, and broaden the base of providers who know what to do. Nutrition science is a century old at least, but how to use it in practice is what families and providers need help understanding. Here's why that gap exists, and how to be successful in spite of it, with your existing provider team. While some nutrition care measures can be done at home on your own, others require professional guidance and input. Reliable, local resources are a great thing to have, as your child may need refinement of nutrition-related assessment and treatments.

The Big Gap

At the 2006 annual conference for the American Dietetic Association, I attended a lecture called "Nutrition Management in Pediatric Rehabilitation." It described standards and goals of nutrition care for infants and children with traumatic brain injuries, stroke, or spinal cord injuries. It did not surprise me that these children have a lot of the same problems as children with autism: cognitive and communication impairments, GI concerns, low muscle tone, gross and fine motor problems, sensory processing handicaps, special nutrition needs, seizures, feeding difficulties. What did surprise me was the degree to which brain-injured children are not only cared for, but loved and embraced by our medical culture—a stark contrast to what children with autism receive when seeking GI or nutrition care. Listening to the hospital staff that gave the presentation, I found myself envious of the clinical attention these unfortunate children get without question, not to mention the support parents receive from bereavement counselors, hospital chaplains, or social service staff, all covered by insurance. Most children in my caseload have an autism spectrum diagnosis. They, too, need an entourage of therapists and providers. I would be thrilled to refer the children I meet for just a fraction of these services, which simply do help children recover, and help their families through it. Clinically speaking, these two groups have many similarities, but they have had very different paths to being in a situation that warrants this care. One group had injuries: skateboard crashes, falls off bikes, near drownings, or strokes. They were injured. What about the other group, the ones with autism? That debate is still at a full boil. Were they injured, or were they born this way?

It shouldn't matter. There is a gap in our medical landscape today for children with autism, in terms of the nutrition and GI piece. They usually can't access this kind of care, even though, clinically speaking, there are valid similarities between children with brain injuries and children with autism spectrum disorders. The lecture I mention here touted supplementation and special nutrition supports for brain-injured children. They benefit from coordinated GI care, physical and occupational therapies, and nutrition care. So do children with autism. This is not to debate whether autism is a brain injury; it is about providing appropriate, ethical treatment for the kinds of problems kids with autism have. The autism epidemic has triggered a deeper search for treatments for neurological conditions and chronic disease. Experience from practice in other areas of conventional medicine—such as pediatric rehabilitation from traumatic brain injuries—and newer pieces from the functional medicine movement, are wending their way into the universe of mainstream providers who help children with autism. Even though this is happening too fast for medical science loyalists and too slow for desperate parents, it is progress.

For many professionals who have served the autism community for a long time, these ideas are not exactly welcome. Ideas that shake the bedrock of anything rarely are. Many parents feel uncomfortable, too, when they bring up whether or not to use a special diet measure with doctors, psychiatrists, psychologists, or neurologists. So far, on balance, pediatricians are not talking much to parents on the use of special diets. They are not recommending them, and not guiding parents who make the decision to use them anyway. This leaves families of affected children in a big gap, a void, which is filled by searching for distant providers who are willing to help, surfing the Net for supplements, protocols, lab tests, and support groups, and bankrupting themselves by paying for all this care out of pocket. Imagine a young snowboarder sustaining a life-changing traumatic brain injury, and the parent then having to search desperately for care, paying for it all, prioritizing all the interventions, discerning which is best, with no input, referral, follow-up, or guidance from a primary care physician, no local services, and no coordination among specialists. This is the common dilemma for families of children with autism spectrum disorders.

When a pediatrician is concerned that one of his young patients may have autism or other learning and developmental delays, he does not make a referral for nutrition care. There are many reasons for this, and it is not because the science behind therapeutic nutrition is weak. Knowing these reasons can help you proceed confidently with your conviction to use a special diet for your child, which by the way is well grounded in decades of nutrition science. Knowing why pediatricians and other MDs in the autism landscape are slow to get on board can also help you engage them in your child's care, which is important for a better outcome. A new dialogue between parent and provider is the offshoot. We are embarking on health care for the most disabled generation of children in U.S. history, so it is time for some serious teamwork, and thorough review of what we are doing. Parents are taking a lead role more than ever before as they seek partnerships with inquisitive providers, rather than the paternal style of pediatric care provided for previous generations. Here are explanations for why there is debate about using special diets as therapy for children with autism. As you will see throughout this book, it is not for lack of good science—but more about history, some holes and gaps in the care delivery landscape, and controversy over what tools are best for children.

Why the Gap Exists:
History, Holes, and Controversy

For nearly a century, Western medicine has understood a lot about the nutritional biochemistry and physiology that create growth, development, and learning in infants and children. So, knowledge about nutrition as a therapeutic tool is not new. The new part is recognizing that kids with autism and other developmental or learning problems often have undiagnosed malabsorption or bowel problems, inadequate diets, or all of the above. We already know that these will impede learning, growth, behavior, and functioning in all children, not just kids with autism—which means that fixing these problems is all the more crucial for a child with a developmental delay or special challenge. Oddly, this is not much applied in pediatrics nowadays—that's the gap. How has this gap been able to widen, much less begin growing in the first place, since autism was first described in the 1940s?

Three reasons: One, history. Autism was given a peculiar set of assumptions and biases created by the first clinicians who encountered it decades ago. Two, holes. These biases managed to stick for decades in large measure due to holes in the training of physicians. In the latter part of the twentieth century, pediatrics, and medicine in general, moved farther and farther away from nutrition and integrative perspectives. Instead, emphasis grew on using pharmaceuticals for symptomatic treatment, and on practice specializations that splintered patients into separate body parts. This model made it acceptable to compartmentalize autism as a disease of the brain only. Three, controversy. The use of special diets for a condition such as autism has been burned into the public consciousness in part by a controversial figure who dared to raise concerns about the single most sacred cow in modern health sciences: vaccines. Put these three reasons together, and it means that most MD providers practicing today in the realm of autism won't go near this special diet stuff, unless they've made a difficult choice to jump the fence and join thousands of parents who just want help. For a doctor, this can mean losing your job, losing your credibility, losing regular income from health insurers who dictate how you practice or prescribe, and starting up your own practice in which you expect families to pay out of pocket.

Physicians are trained to regard autism and other learning or developmental diagnoses as brain problems, not whole body problems. Findings about gut or nutrition problems are too new to be incorporated into anybody's training. And most MDs don't study nutrition anyway—their training and practice are focused on pharmaceutical approaches. Lastly, and surely not least, is the mention of vaccines as anything but miraculous. This can clear a room fast (or perhaps fill it fast, depending on which side of the debate you've fallen). Let's take a quick look at these three pitfalls your provider may have hit, in supporting your goals and interest in using a special diet.

History: The Dark Ages

Autism was first described in the 1940s. Regarded as a psychiatric condition, it had no precedent in the medical literature before then.* Some of the very first cases ever described included comments on extreme feeding and nutrition issues, but these were regarded as meaningless peculiarities. The odd bowel problems, violent or aggressive behavior after eating, and bizarre self-imposed diet restrictions garnered little attention, other than to be assumed just another of autism's weird psychological features. The children were believed to be incapable of love, communication, connection, or emotion. Hence the now thankfully defunct phrase "refrigerator mothers," which referred to the belief that some mothers were emotionally so frozen, they could not love and care for their children, and this caused autism.

This stunning conclusion held sway as the bedrock of truth under autism. It kept curiosity about the physiology of autism to essentially zero for decades. As incredible as that is, remnants of this thinking linger even today. As recently as 2004, a parent reported to me that the neurologist who diagnosed her toddler at a highly respected children's medical center in New England gave this news: "Your child has

---

*Some note Pink's Disease, which appeared before 1920, as the first mention of anything autism-like. It was linked to a mercury-containing teething powder popular in the early twentieth century. Mercury was withdrawn from this and other baby products by 1948, but it remains in some vaccines today.

autism. He will never love you, or be capable of loving you. Don't waste your time loving him, and in fact, you should start now to distance yourself from him. Stop hugging him; he doesn't understand."

This is so profoundly wrong, hopeless, and devastating that it leaves me speechless. I shared this with an in-house colleague of the neurologist and was assured that corrective action would be taken. I have never encountered a parent who believed this about his or her affected child. All parents relate moments, even if they are precious few, of affection, recognition, and love with their children affected by autism. This is the type of provider to simply drop like a stone, and walk away. Save your energy for those who will support you.

Holes: The Nutrition Disconnect in Modern Pediatrics

In spite of solid science on how child nutrition drives development, learning, and growth, a disconnect prevails in medicine today that goes something like this: Sure, kids need good nutrition to grow. But what does that have to do with the brain? And anyway, if nutrition were a big enough problem to injure the brains of kids with developmental or learning disorders, then surely these kids would not grow normally. Kids have to have adequate diets, and healthy intestines to absorb those diets, in order to grow. They're growing, so nutrition is not part of the picture, and there is thus no link between diets, absorption, and what is going on in their brains. Right? Wrong.

You may have a chorus of providers telling you something along those lines, or that there is no proof that special diets help children with autism, Asperger's, sensory processing disorder, or other learning and developmental issues. The nutrition piece of the autism puzzle is easy for these providers to miss, and misunderstand. This doesn't mean it is not valid. This means they missed it, because they don't study nutrition, don't do nutrition assessment and monitoring, and don't implement therapeutic diets. Dietitians and nutritionists do that, not psychiatrists, psychologists, neurologists, or pediatricians. Without a referral to a dietitian from one of these providers, you're probably not going to find one. Even if you did, she is probably working in a major medical center with a mixed-nuts caseload of everything under the sun. She does not have the time or freedom to specialize in therapeutic diets for learning and developmental disorders, especially when the physicians above her in her workplace don't consider it a relevant tool.

Here's what we typically find in these kids, once the right provider takes a thoughtful look: Emerging research shows they usually do have bowel issues and nutrition problems. Children with autism have bowel symptoms more often than typical peers. They feel better and function better when these are treated. Up to 80 percent of children with autism may have active bowel symptoms, including reflux, constipation, chronic loose stool, bloating, or gas (who can learn to potty train with all that going on?). Upwards of half of affected children assessed further for GI concerns show changes in tissue throughout the throat, stomach, and intestines, from ulcers and inflamed bumpy tissue ("cobbled" or "nodular" tissue), to blunted villous tips, to eosinophilic infiltration in the GI tract (eosinophils are white blood cells associated with allergy). This can be painful; how does a nonverbal child tell you? Like coral in a healthy reef, villi are the delicate tips in the small intestine that absorb nutrients from digested food moving past. If they are flattened, they're broken, and they are not absorbing nutrients well, if at all. This can be occurring with no obvious bowel symptoms, with mild GI symptoms, or with obvious GI symptoms. Either way, it can profoundly affect behavior, learning, attention, or sensory modulation.

Even for pediatricians who are poking, measuring, and talking to kids every day, red flags for these problems easily fly under the radar. Pediatricians meet some cursory requirements in nutrition, but several have intimated to me that they know little about it and are grateful for input. A nutrition assessment is not part of a typical pediatric visit, nor is it a pediatrician's job to perform one. It takes too long. Some data show the average time spent by a pediatrician with parents at routine visits is less than five minutes. So that means your child can come and go from the pediatrician a lot, and no one will be the wiser that there may be a nutrition problem—it never gets assessed. Even if a problem is suspected, nutrition tools are not what most pediatricians grab from their treatment toolbox. Prescription drugs are usually the treatment of first and only resort—despite findings that homeopathic and simple nutritional changes can work as well or better, without side effects. Unfortunately, the typical pediatrician doesn't know about these simple, safe alternatives, unless he or she has taken special pains to study what conventional medical wisdom dismisses as poorly proven.

Here's an anecdote to illustrate this point: I have met a number of toddlers placed on growth hormone injections. These are children who stopped growing, or slowed down their growth so much that they fell below the 5th percentile for height or weight for age. Even in these cases, no nutrition referrals were made by their pediatric MD providers. Endocrinology referrals were; an assumption was made that an esoteric problem such as hormone chemistry, not diets or gut health, caused the children to experience growth failure. I find this astounding. Would we not prefer to rule out the simple stuff first? In each of these cases I encountered, the children had never been given a nutrition assessment, never were screened for inflammation from foods, and were never regarded in terms of what might be disrupting absorption. In each case, I found gliadin (gluten) sensitivity, fungal overgrowth in the bowel, and poor food intakes. In each case, the children began growing again when these nutritional issues were treated. They did not need growth hormone injections. This is how modern medicine wanders from common sense, low-tech options, and toward what is lucrative for a corporate health landscape or intriguing for the bench biochemist.

Besides not implementing nutrition tools, pediatricians may not notice the subtle growth shifts that often show up for children with developmental and learning diagnoses. Though subtle, these can yield some great clues about how to use a special diet. As for how children grow when they have autism, the more we look, the more we notice some differences. Boys with Asperger's syndrome, for example, tend to have a body mass index (BMI) that is below healthy levels (too thin for their height). This places them at nutritional risk: A too-low BMI is associated with more frequent illness and infection, and more cognitive/attention problems. Meanwhile, children with classic autism often show unusually large head circumference with robust growth along weight and height percentiles. Does this mean they are more likely to be obese—now a major public health issue for U.S. children? One study found that kids with autism were not obese more often than typical peers. Still, they may be at higher risk, since participating in sports and athletics is exceptionally challenging for many kids on the spectrum. Studies on children with food allergies, now far more prevalent than twenty years ago and more common in children with autism, suggest that they have poorer intakes for certain nutrients and may not grow as well as typical peers. Food allergies and sensitivities are yet another piece seen more often in kids with autism that makes eating and absorbing an adequate diet even harder.

In my own practice, I often see departures from expected growth patterns in children with autism, Asperger's, or ADHD. I find them when pediatricians don't, simply because I am free to take extra time to regard several growth parameters together with food intake data. A routine pediatric visit will usually check your child's weight and height for age. These do not provide a full assessment of your child's growth status, according to the American Dietetic Association's 2008 publication on pediatric nutrition assessment. Body mass index (BMI), weight to height ratio, head circumference for kids up to age two or three, weight and height for age, birth weight and length, and pattern of growth from birth are all relevant to assessing a child's growth pattern and status. I also routinely calculate a child's percent of ideal body weight and height-age equivalent. Who cares? I do, because when all this is juxtaposed with food intake data, it reveals a lot about what is awry with a child's gut, whether growth is truly progressing as it should, and if the brain is getting a short shrift on nutrients and energy. There is simply no time for all this in most pediatricians' offices today: Visit duration is predetermined by your insurance company or by the doctor's HMO employer, not by the doctor.

Controversy: The Sacred Cow

The vaccine controversy is often the elephant in the room around special diet conversations, and it has fractured communication between many families and their providers. Knowing a little about this may help you avoid a breakdown between you and people you need on your child's care team. In the 1990s, some researchers began asking if autism (and all its lighter variants) is a gut disease and a brain disease in one—a whole body condition rather than a brain problem. Before the mercury story ever got legs, the idea that some sort of newly noted bowel disease may drive features of autism was introduced in 1998. These findings stunned the medical community worldwide. They were a resounding quake to autism's bedrock. They rapidly increased interest in special diets, because gluten (wheat) intolerance emerged as a side effect of the damage found in intestines of the children with autism who were studied. It had been documented for nearly a century that when diets are poor or absorption is impaired, then developmental delay, growth problems, learning problems, and frequent infections or even death from infectious disease are expected outcomes. Though nobody would deny that infants and children require normal absorption of healthy diets to grow, learn, and develop, linking a bowel disease to a developmental impairment seemed far-fetched.

Part of the mystery in autism may be in the absorption part. The

1998 findings described such progressed, distinct disease in the intestines of these children that typical absorption of their diets was impossible. It was a new type of bowel disease. It did not match conditions such as Crohn's disease, celiac disease, or ulcerative colitis. What was it? It was given the descriptive term "autistic enterocolitis," then after more investigation and publication "ileal lymphoid nodular hyperplasia," which is another way of saying badly inflamed, bumpy, swollen intestinal tissue that, so far, has been seen only in children with autism. It was obviously a painful condition that the affected children could not understand, much less verbalize to their parents. It wasn't rare. It occurred in too many of the children with autism assessed.

This touched off a storm of controversy. Regarding what was assumed to be a psychiatric disorder as a biological disease was unheard of. The medical community was reluctant to acknowledge these children had any type of bowel disease, much less a previously unknown variant that might yield clues to autism treatment or causes. Many pediatric gastroenterologists are hesitant today to fully assess children with autism, because they do not want scrutiny and controversy. They may not fully understand these findings if they have read of them only through the filter of the media. This is important for parents to know, because it explains why it is still difficult for children with autism spectrum challenges to get adequately screened and treated for GI problems.

While this work was applauded by thousands of families whose children benefited from it, medical officials decried it. Aside from postulating that a bowel disease so early in life might affect the brain, the real problem was mentioning that these children appeared to stop being typically developing, typically eating, and typically pooping toddlers when they received their measles-mumps-rubella (MMR) vaccinations. Some stopped growing normally; all began having severe bowel symptoms and feeding problems that they had never had. Insidiously more than with a singular crash, as the weird bowel signs and self-imposed diet restrictions emerged in these children, they also slid backward developmentally, losing communication skill, losing social reference, losing motor skills, and acquiring bizarre anxieties and perseverations after this shot. By now, many thousands of parents are familiar with this story, while many providers still find it beyond unbelievable.

When more study found the DNA of vaccine strain measles in the gut tissue of children with autism, controversy exploded all the more. Further clinical trials in other locations were halted, ostensibly to prevent panic and keep parents' confidence in vaccination high. But the DNA findings suggested that this never-seen-before viral infection in the intestines of children with autism was possibly from the MMR vaccine. It did not come from a wild measles strain, which has a different DNA profile. And it had no business infecting gut tissue in any case. Its presence there begged the question of whether the virus also infected brain tissue in affected children, a pertinent question, since for sixty years we have accepted that in utero or very early viral infections can be a trigger for mental retardation. This finding implied a problem with this vaccine for a subset of children, and touched off the controversy that most of us have heard about by now.

That tale has now been told, retold, and spun with every possible slant for a decade. Parents who delay or defer vaccinations because of it have been widely vilified (which does not make much sense; the vaccines are meant to defend against infection, so the vast number of adults and children who have received them should not be at risk). What has received less attention is that an MMR vaccine would not be an entirely implausible trigger for inflammatory bowel disease. It was already known that getting viral infections repeatedly or in close succession appeared to trigger bowel diseases, and that some people were more susceptible than others. No one thought this work to be controversial. The route of exposure—a vaccine—was different in the autism cases, but it was a clustered viral exposure nonetheless. Saying that the route of exposure to the clustered viral material was a vaccine became the flash point. Enter the sacred cow of our medical culture.

Is there a more volatile topic between you and your pediatrician than the question of when, if, or how to vaccinate? If your child has autism, you need to know if inflammatory bowel disease is part of the struggle. Whether vaccinations have acted as a trigger may impact your child's success with nutrition care. Even when present to a milder degree, gut inflammation can be painful and it will interfere with learning, growth, and development. There are treatments for it. You will find answers in this book about what you can do at home about it, and what you can ask of your providers. Not all children with autism have bowel disease this severe, but most appear to have treatable nutrition and GI problems. These are problems that get treated with little fanfare in typically developing children. We can also treat them in children with autism spectrum challenges, sensory dysregulation, or attention and learning problems.

What can parents do if their providers are less than inquisitive on the child's behalf? See the resources section for gastroenterology findings in autism, and share the peer-reviewed material with your provider. For children needing GI care, be persistent. Find a doctor who will work with you, and be curious about how to restore your child's health. If your child is not improving under his care, point this out, and initiate a discussion about what the next reasonable measures should be. If your GI provider has only been willing to prescribe Miralax or Prevacid, or medications that mask symptoms without looking at what triggers symptoms, you should ask why other methods have not been considered. Medicating constipation or reflux has its place, but it does not correct why these problems occur in the first place. Some of these drugs are not ideal to use indefinitely. Begin a discussion with your provider about new strategies, and bring the articles listed in "Resources and Further Reading" for your MD provider to review. A physician's job is to be a curious and effective clinician.

How to Engage a Reluctant Provider . . .
and When Simply to Move On

If your doctor is not on board with your interest in nutrition supports for your child, you might succeed with a few tactful efforts at bridging the gap. Many parents with children affected by autism spectrum issues have sought specialists in other states to guide care. Some families are comfortable with a geographically distant doctor for the complex care of a child with autism. While their expertise in biomedical treatment tools is needed, so are your local mainstream providers. Build your local network by assigning reasonable expectations to the providers capable of helping with different facets of your child's care. You may need them in an emergency. For the most part, these are people who want to do a good job. They are in an unprecedented position at the moment: Families are demanding a service they know little about, or questioning a basic component of their training. Before you start special diet measures, see the professional learning module on this topic in the resources section and consider sharing it with your child's pediatrician, neurologist, gastroenterologist, or whomever you'd like to read it. The more peer review on this that physicians can read, the easier it may be for them to help.

Some physicians relish the authority role of old, while others are more open to new strategies that respect parents and include them in decisions. As they are all simply human, they may well respond to the olive branch being extended. If not, move on to a different provider. Because I have unfortunately received many stories of what might be winnable in a court as medical negligence or misconduct, I make these two recommendations: A provider who obstructs your every effort to seek improvements for your child is probably never going to get on your team. Verbally abusive doctors should be reported to their state licensure board. A pediatrician who permits a child to languish in poor nutrition status (that is, a child who loses weight or stops growing) while making no referral for appropriate care or while offering no measures to correct this is medically negligent, and this should be reported, too. Barring these egregious conduct issues, trust your instincts on how to proceed with your child's providers.

These are conundrums parents do not expect. My husband and I found our pediatric group so unable to guide us that we dropped them before our son was seven months old. We chose to work instead with a pediatric family nurse practitioner who specialized in classical homeopathy. This was very successful for treating infections, illnesses, and small emergencies, and for improving our son's developmental progress. We also switched his primary provider over to our family practice physician, whom we had known for years and felt we could trust. We patched together a network that eventually included these providers as well as a naturopathic doctor, specialists in developmental pediatrics at our region's major children's medical center, and a pediatric occupational therapist. The point is, you will need to assemble a team that works for you. Find providers you like and trust. You are the boss of the team, so find people who will work with you, not against you. If you don't like your pediatrician, there are many others—and other types of health care professionals—to explore. Meanwhile, here are some conversation tools that may help keep a good but reluctant provider in your corner, if you would like to discuss using a special diet or nutrition measure:

- "I would like your help and support, because we value you as our primary provider. I know these tools are unfamiliar and you want to do the right thing. Could we agree to try this out for six months?"
- "What would be your concerns with using special diets and nutrition measures? I want to be sure we approach them correctly."

- "Let's try this for six months, and agree on the rules. What are the red flags I should know about that signal trouble for my child while using a special diet?"

- Would you take a look at this lab test I have heard about, so we can consider its benefits together? I would like to try it, and I hope I can have your input."

- "I'm wondering what your opinion would be on this peer-reviewed literature about using special diets. I found it helpful but it is written for health professionals, and I would value your guidance on how I can use this."

- "We are going forward with some diet and nutrition tools, and I would very much value your guidance. What are your concerns or ideas?"

- "I'm concerned about my child's nutrition status, because his diet is so limited. What supplements should I add? How can I improve his diet? Can you refer me to someone familiar with using special diets or nutrition care for children with these issues?"

- "What have other parents in your practice done for special diets?"

- "I'm interested in gluten-free to start. Can you refer me to a local celiac support group or organization, or a provider familiar with going gluten-free?"

- "My child is still not potty trained and we have tried everything else. Humor me, and let us try antifungal therapy. I have heard that it helps children with bowel incontinence in some cases. What do you think?"

- "I'm wondering if my child would benefit from a special diet. Would you be willing to work with us on this?" If not: "Can you refer me to someone who can help? I want to be sure we do this safely and effectively. Would you be willing to communicate with that provider?"

Closing the Gap, Getting to Work

Though pediatricians and pediatric MD specialists do not typically make a close study of nutrition science and practice, they can acknowledge basic facts about children, growth, and development relative to it. Rather than starting with a debate about vaccine safety, work from the common turf you have with your provider: Children need to be in normal nutrition status to learn, grow, and develop typically. Express your concerns for your child's food intake if it is poor or overly restricted, the growth pattern if there are problems, or ask for help in testing for problems with absorption if growth or bowel symptoms are active. This will mean you are asking for referrals, which your pediatrician may not know how to make for the kinds of questions you are asking. Be direct, and respectful. If no referral is forthcoming, ask the pediatrician to guide you, letting him know you plan to proceed anyway. If all else fails, let him know you are willing to keep him informed of your child's progress and revisit opportunities to get his input. In whatever way that works, expanding your provider resources is your goal, so that you are not alone on the Internet searching for protocols and ordering lab tests. If you have a biomedical provider you like in another state, see if progress notes can be shared between this provider and your local pediatrician.

Finding an Expert

Because this is a new, rapidly emerging area of care for children, your pediatrician may be ill equipped to help you with special diets as a therapy for your child. Engaging her in the process is a good idea, and you can learn together. But what if you would like to find someone who has trod this path many times before? There are no accredited university programs for this genre yet, but a steadfast rule is to work with licensed health care providers. Keep a clear line of distinction between supportive parents, chat groups, websites, and listservs on the one hand, and true medical care on the other. Naturopathic doctors, MDs, family nurse practitioners, and nutrition professionals are licensed to practice in their respective disciplines and have jumped through many hoops to get and keep their licenses, so that patients get responsible, safe, and appropriate care. If you have reservations about their guidance, bring your questions to them, so your child can get the most from their training and experience.

What Licensure in Nutrition Means for Your Child

Nutrition professionals are licensed in all but six states. Like any other health professional, nutritionists you work with should be licensed. Two things that a licensed dietitian or nutritionist can offer your child are enhanced access to insurance coverage for nutrition care, and appropriate monitoring of growth and nutrition status. Licensure for nutritionists is a rigorous credential that requires at least one accredited university degree in a nutrition or health sciences discipline, as well as hundreds of hours of supervised training in clinic settings. In some states, it may require registration status with the American Dietetic Association as well, which in itself has stiff requirements for university degrees in approved curricula and supervised training. It then requires passing a lengthy exam akin to medical boards for a doctor, or a bar exam for a lawyer. Licensure also requires proof of continuing education with ongoing, accredited coursework. Naturopaths, chiropractors, osteopaths, and medical doctors are also subject to professional licensure, just like nutritionists/dietitians. Providers often pursue and maintain an out-of-state license if they live where licensure laws are not yet enacted, as they should.

Licensed providers of nutrition care can bill insurance for nutrition services or, at the very least, can code your care appropriately, so that insurance is more likely to cover it. A licensed nutritionist or dietitian is the provider that health insurers expect to reimburse or pay when it comes to nutrition care. Your insurance company is probably not going to pay a neurologist for nutrition service such as prescribing a special diet, any more than they would reimburse me for providing a neurological evaluation (which I have no business doing). They also are unlikely to pay a provider with mysterious credentials for any service. Choose providers who are adequately trained for your child's needs, who are licensed in their profession, and who are providing service in their discipline, not someone else's.

The other piece that a nutrition provider should provide for your child is assessment and monitoring. Licensure requirements for nutrition professionals include training in nutrition assessment and monitoring for children, while those for other disciplines do not. For example, an individual with a PhD in a nutrition discipline may be learned in cellular chemistry relative to nutrients, but will usually have no training to actually work with patients of any age, let alone infants and children. Assessment and monitoring is essential for nutrition care in children. It means using clinical standards for careful tracking of a child's growth pattern, total food intake, and nutrition signs and symptoms. Most children in my caseload have begun using special diets before I meet them. What I frequently find is that their diets have not been adequate to support growth and learning. Their diets have either ceased being therapeutically effective, or are actually detrimental, because no one kept tabs on basics like growth progress or actual food intakes.

Who should do the nutritionist's job and how is a line that gets blurred a lot, with all the best intentions, in the Defeat Autism Now (DAN) community. Through conference trainings, the DAN community is actively reaching out to give professionals information they need to help children on the spectrum. Psychiatrists, neurologists, and MDs or nurses in all kinds of disciplines have become "DAN providers" and offer their services for special diets, chelation, supplements, and medications to families affected by autism. The great part about this is that many children are on their way to much improved functioning with these tools. The lousy part is that since these professionals are providing a service outside their disciplines, insurance companies may not cover the care. This is truly a shame as it makes this care out of reach for so many children. Try these measures to access this care under insurance:

- If you have a DAN provider now and the care is not covered, check that your provider is using nutrition care diagnosis and procedure codes on your billing statements. Psychiatric codes do not trigger reimbursement for nutrition services. See "Resources and Further Reading" for nutrition codes that may apply for your child.
- Work with a licensed nutrition professional who is also a registered dietitian, if possible—simply because insurance companies recognize these credentials as applicable for nutrition care. Use nutrition diagnosis and procedure codes that apply for your child.
- Get a written referral or a referral number from your pediatrician for nutrition care (a verbal okay usually doesn't fly with insurance companies). This is valid whenever there are concerns for your child's growth pattern, food intake, or nutrition status, or if your child is getting sick frequently.
- Don't ask for or accept a written referral under a diagnosis code for autism, when you are planning to work with a provider on nutrition and special diets. The diagnosis code under which the referral is made should reflect nutrition concerns, not developmental concerns, in order for the insurance company to consider it. For example, it should say

"moderate calorie malnutrition" (263.0) or "mineral metabolism disorder NOS" (275.9) or "allergic colitis" (558.9). Your provider should use the code most descriptive of the nutrition condition; there are dozens to choose from. Your child's referral or treatment should not be coded under autism codes (299.01).

- Insurance companies will probably not pay for nutrition care with an individual who bills solely under a PhD credential, such as a psychologist or a nutritional biochemist, or providers who don't have a license to practice nutrition care. Some insurers may pay other licensed providers (MDs, NDs) if appropriate coding is used. Insurers do not reimburse individuals who don't have appropriate degrees to practice.

Adding a licensed nutrition professional to your team will also plug in the growth and food intakes monitoring piece that is often missing from the DAN providers' protocols (if that's not possible, your DAN provider can use the accredited learning module on this—see the resources section). DAN practitioner trainings are fantastic for presenting the latest biochemistry updates for autism spectrum disorders, but they do not confer or require degrees or licensure in a health sciences discipline. Unlicensed individuals can become DAN practitioners, as can providers licensed in areas that do not require clinical training in pediatrics or child nutrition. Because children with autism spectrum concerns so often have nutrition and GI problems, good nutrition assessment and monitoring is critical for them. Special diets do work, but they need monitoring with the right provider team to be safe and to reach their potential for success. If your child is not progressing as you expect, ask your providers what to do about it. Another provider's point of view may help. With so many layers to assess and address, kids on the spectrum benefit from a team approach.

A Final Word About Vaccines

Most families I meet who are interested in nutrition tools for their children's developmental diagnoses have questions about this. They are valid questions, since I have observed booster doses of vaccines to delay or reverse progress with nutrition care. If there is a problem with our vaccination schedule, the sooner we know, the better. The former head of the Institute of Medicine (IOM) at the National Institutes of Health (NIH), Bernadine Healy, MD, announced in May 2008 that review of vaccines as a trigger for autism was too quickly swept under the rug by herself and her colleagues. For her, many of her peers in practice, and tens of thousands of families, it is not a closed debate.

Pediatricians usually fervently believe that full compliance with the vaccination schedule is best. There is plenty of pressure on parents to comply. Why do parents have such persistent concerns? Aside from the autism controversy, other pediatric conditions have risen with the increase in vaccinations given. The United States uses more vaccines than any other country in the world, but has an infant mortality rate worse than nearly thirty other countries and some of the highest rates of chronic disease in children. One in six of our children is learning disabled; one in nine has asthma; one in 150 has autism; one in 450 has diabetes. All of these conditions have risen dramatically since 1980, when the vaccine schedule became more crowded. Ninety-five percent of all six-year-olds are fully vaccinated in the United States, with dozens of recommended doses of vaccine. Parents today are in an unprecedented quandary, wondering how to approach the demand to use so many vaccines on their children. This topic has fractured communication between countless families and their pediatricians, a relationship that we would all prefer to see intact.

Many parents are unaware that they do have control over this facet of a child's health care. Learn about your rights, which vary by state. Don't be caught off guard without your chosen course of action when the first needle comes out. During family planning and pregnancy is a good time to sort out these choices, not during labor and delivery or at your first well-baby checkup. As your child will be expected to take boosters repeatedly throughout childhood and even when entering college, you will need to refresh your information often. Find a provider who respects curiosity about this hotly debated issue. Some parents choose to spread vaccinations out and give fewer doses at a time, rather than nine or twelve in a single visit, as is frequently done in the United States today. Some parents choose to defer some vaccines while allowing others. Still others are eager to learn about naturopathic immune supports or homeopathic tools, which work well for childhood infections and illness. These are not tools your pediatrician is trained to use, so don't look there for a glowing opinion or guidance on how to use them. In that case, parents should work with experienced pediatric homeopaths (look for a classical homeopath) or licensed naturopathic doctor, rather than prescribe for their own children unassisted. Some MD providers are happy to work with professionals in these other modalities, some are not, and some may earn additional credentials themselves to use these tools in conjunction with conventional medicine, which can also work well. There are many reasonable choices, and the more information gathered, the healthier your child will be. The objective is just that: good health, normal development, a contented child.

Nutrition Therapies and Special Diets Are Effective . . . No Matter Where You Stand in the Debate

The debates will continue about whether vaccines can trigger autism in a subset of children, about the studies claiming to either refute or support this theory, or whether the original researchers should share a

Nobel Prize or go to jail. Every study, clinical trial, case review, or parent anecdote relating to the biomedical treatment model and diets for special-needs kids will be picked apart, blogged, criticized, and/or lauded for a long time to come. There are now hundreds, perhaps thousands, of peer-reviewed published reports, and even more anecdotes; it will take years. There may never be a conclusive answer that satisfies everyone, and there is no need to wait for one. We already know how to help children when it comes to nutrition care. Whether a child has diabetes, asthma, traumatic brain injury, leukemia, cystic fibrosis, growth failure, measles, autism, or learning disabilities, good nutrition support and medical nutrition therapy are safe, reliable components of their total health care plan.

Strong nutrition status in children is arguably the single most important factor for normal, effective, vigorous, and successful immune response to infectious disease. Recovering from an illness such as chickenpox or measles is routine in children who are in solid nutrition status. Children in poor nutrition status have complications, longer illness, or death from infectious disease more often than their healthy counterparts. Facets of child nutrition, such as status for protein, growth, or vitamins and minerals, can make or break the outcome of an infectious disease.

For children with chronic conditions and disabilities, strong nutrition status is all the more crucial. With the numbers of children facing an autism diagnosis projected into the millions in the next decade, and other chronic conditions in children doubled and tripled in a generation, anything that enhances abilities for these children is a must-do measure. Nutrition status is the first layer, the most important layer, and the foundation for other needed therapies and treatments for all children.

Once that foundation is restored, the more esoteric pieces you may have heard about can be tapped with greater success, may be needed to a lesser extent or for a shorter course, or may not be needed at all. Chelation, methylcobalamin nasal spray, spironolactone, glutathione, intravenous immunoglobulin, vitamin A therapy, antiviral therapy, hyperbaric oxygen therapy, therapeutic listening, occupational therapy, applied behavior analysis—this is just a partial list of the myriad therapies in use for children with special needs along the autism spectrum. Good primary nutrition assessment and monitoring helps you prioritize which of these treatments your child might need, and when to use them for maximum benefit.

Meanwhile, as you set out to assemble your team, there are strategies for special diets and nutrition supports that can start at home. How to begin and how to follow a reliably successful sequence of nutrition care are described in the next chapter. Consider these professionals for your rotation of go-to providers. You won't need all of them all the time, but building relationships across a network of helpers who are willing to communicate with each other and you creates a net around your child to support optimal growth, learning, and development.

- **Pediatrician.** This is your local emergency contact, provider of referrals, communicator to specialists about your child, and first point of access for insurance-covered care.
- **Naturopathic doctor (licensed).** Find one with ample experience with pediatric patients. This is your resource for gentle, safe ways to support your child's immune function and GI needs with non-pharmacological tools, and for access to novel lab diagnostics that your pediatrician may not know about. School physicals can be obtained with an ND, if vaccine questions become too contentious with your pediatrician.
- **Gastroenterologist.** This provider will assess degree of bowel disease in cases where signs and symptoms warrant it. Your GI provider can help you consider medications for inflammation, reflux, imbalanced bowel flora (see Chapter 3), or poor appetite, or can help you access specialized formulas that may help your child (see Chapter 5). Some children need

bowel impactions treated as well and your GI doctor can do this too.

- **Neurologist.** If your child has a seizure disorder, this provider can inform on medication options and order diagnostics like brain scans if pertinent.
- **Therapists for speech, language, occupational, physical, or sensory integration therapies.** These people will provide long-term, much-needed repetitious therapies that engage areas of the brain frequently challenged in autism and other disabilities.
- **Licensed nutrition professional.** If nutrition assessment and monitoring is not done by the naturopath or pediatrician, this person can ensure that your child's special diet is safe, adequate, and effective enough to support expected growth and development.
- **DAN providers.** If you have no support forthcoming on your in-network or local provider landscape, interview several providers who use DAN techniques (see www.autism.com for a list of DAN providers). Look for eight to ten years' experience (ask "When did you attend your first DAN training?"), success stories that you can speak to personally, and ask about policies for payment in advance. See Chapter 3 for more on how DAN providers use lab data in treatment plans. DAN providers who are licensed health professionals (MDs, NDs, family nurse practitioners, or dietitians/nutritionists) are preferable, because they have had standardized training in university and clinical settings prior to DAN.
- **Psychologists, psychiatrists, licensed social workers.** These individuals can use therapies to support your child outside of nutrition tools, can identify your child's needs for school settings, can attend school meetings in some cases to help advocate for your child's needs, and can refine developmental diagnoses. They can also support your child with medication choices.

TWO

Nutrition Therapy 101

The Essential Steps to Take, Terms to Know, and Principles to Understand

Individualized Nutrition Is Best

Special diets and supplements for children with issues such as autism spectrum disorders, sensory integration disorder, ADHD, or learning and behavioral diagnoses have been popular for several years, but there is yet to be a consensus on what works best. I don't expect there ever will be—not because therapeutic nutrition measures are ineffective, but because nutrition care must be *individualized* to work best. If a particular psychiatric medication does not help a child with ADHD, we do not say that all psych meds do not help any children. We move through a process that identifies what would work best for that child, and so it goes for nutrition care. There is no one special diet, or one biomedical protocol, that works for all kids. The nutrition concerns that take priority might be different for each child, and these need to be individually assessed. If anything is true across the board, it is that nutrition assessment works best in a certain sequence (discussed later in this chapter), even if its findings differ for each child. Unfortunately, providers using these diets who are also knowledgeable about nutrition assessment and monitoring of children with special needs are few and far between right now. That is why working with the licensed and in-network providers you have, as described in the first chapter, is a good idea. Both you and your providers are going to be working as a team and learning together.

By now most readers have heard of the biomedical treatment model for autism. This is a phrase that encompasses all the treatments now in use to correct peculiar physiological features that keep popping up with autism diagnoses. These treatments include special diets, supplements, chelation, hyperbaric oxygen therapy, GI care, and so on. So far, most researchers in the biomedical community concur that autism appears to worsen in severity with worsening immune function, bowel/digestive function, and toxic burden. Nutrition status affects each of these, and nutrition therapies can improve each of these. Individually assessing each layer is important for any child—as long as it is done in a sequence that treats the bottom-most layers first. In practice, I approach the nutrition care process in a sequence that addresses this "lowest" layer first. Some of this is based on Defeat Autism Now (DAN) protocols, which I began learning in 1999. To these, I add established tenets of child nutrition monitoring, standards that have existed in clinical nutrition practice for decades. This strengthens the Defeat Autism Now tools by making sure your child's special diet is safe, adequate, and effective. I have written a course module for health professionals on this, which is listed in the resources section. It is called "Medical Nutrition Therapy for Pediatric Autism: Strategies for Assessment and Monitoring." It is the first peer-reviewed, accredited document to instruct health professionals on how to incorporate standards of child nutrition monitoring, so that special diets can be safer, adequate, and more effective.

If your in-network provider is unfamiliar with how nutrition plays into your child's learning or developmental diagnosis, sharing this module is a good place to start. It can help allay a common concern: Many doctors wonder if special diets for autism are safe or adequate. The truth is, they often are not, based on my own findings in practice assessing children who have used a special diet. Believe it or not, children using these diets under an MD's supervision appear to be no better off than children whose families use the Internet or books for guidance. This is often because no one is monitoring growth or food intakes—the bottom layer for a child. Though they are good at ordering and interpreting lab tests, MD providers are not trained to monitor or implement therapeutic diets. The course module I wrote, which is accredited to give licensed health professionals continuing education credits, can show any interested providers how to monitor special diets safely. Because children with autism spectrum concerns so often show nutrition and GI problems, good nutrition monitoring is critical for them. Special diets do work, but they need monitoring to be safe and adequate, and to reach their potential for success.

There are excellent resources for parents and providers that explain, in great detail, all the shifted physiological layers that have been noticed in children with autism. The list is long, the biochemistry complicated: immune dysregulation and autoimmune problems; compromised digestive function; gut inflammation; unusually high burdens of toxic metals such as mercury or lead; unusually high levels of essential metals such as copper or iron; deficits for other essential minerals such as zinc, magnesium, or selenium; wasting of sulfur, a necessary element for several structural and messenger proteins in the body; florid overgrowth of disruptive bowel bacteria and yeast; viral load that is too high, such as an exceptionally high titer for measles or cytomegalovirus; diminished methylation capacity, something that can impact mood, attention, and detoxification; suppressed ability to excrete toxins or tolerate medications. The level of detail needed to fully explain each of these problem areas is well summarized and referenced in other books, and exhaustively articulated in research articles; see the resources section for suggested reading. Not every child with autism has a problem with every layer, which makes individualized assessment and care all the more important. The focus of this book is to synthesize all that detail into a plan for you at home. What do you do with it all, especially the food part? What lab tests do you really need? How do you get your insurance to cover it? What if your doctor is unsupportive? What foods need to be withdrawn, and how can you tell? What are safe and adequate replacements? What about all these supplements, which ones should you try? At what doses? Is this safe? Starting with that lowest layer—your child's growth pattern and food intakes—prioritizes this for you. This sequence has been successful for me in practice, and you can use it with your providers. Its very first piece takes a close look at one part of your child's nutrition picture that you may think is absolutely fine. Even if it is, I always start with it: growth.

Use These Steps in This Order for Safe and Effective Special Diet Measures

Without getting into every layer of biochemistry pertinent to autism or other learning and developmental concerns, you can use the steps below, in the order suggested here. Leaving any one of these things undone, partly done, or reversing/altering the sequence usually means the special diet intervention does not go as well, in my experience. Because the first step is so crucial to success of the entire special diet intervention, it gets much of this chapter's attention. The steps are:

1. Check your child's basic nutrition status *first*. Whether this is done by you or your provider, this means assuring that your child is growing entirely as expected and his current food intake is adequate (exactly how to do this is discussed later in this chapter). Ideally, do this before special diet measures are

begun. If nutrition status is compromised even a little, this means that some of your child's learning, developmental, or behavior challenges are due to inappropriate total food intake and/or compromised growth status. Fixing these must come early in the special diet plan, or success with other tools such as supplements and chelation will be impeded.

2. Correct bowel flora. Bowel flora are the microbes humans need in the GI tract to help digest and absorb food, and fend off invasive pathogens (viruses, microbial parasites, or detrimental bacteria). Good bowel flora—the helpful bacteria for your gut—keep the lining of the GI tract healthy and keep bowel habits normal. Newborns especially rely on the right bowel bacteria to help them digest first feedings and develop normal immune function. Antibiotics, toxic metal exposures, vaccines, and certain viral or bacterial exposures can disrupt bowel flora.

3. Replace foods that your child doesn't tolerate with foods of equal or better nutritional value. The usual suspects: gluten, casein, soy. Lab studies may or may not be needed to discern exactly which foods are most inflammatory for your child's immune system or GI tract. A common mistake is replacing cow's milk with nutritionally vacant milks made from rice, potato, or almond. While these are suitable for baking or cooking, they are inadequate milk substitutes for children who rely on fluid milk for protein and fats.

4. Replenish micronutrients—that is, vitamins and minerals. Some may be best used at therapeutic (high) doses, some may be fine at typical doses, some may be best used in specific formulations. How to do this depends on clinical signs and symptoms your child is showing, and sometimes on lab studies.

5. Check for signs and symptoms of GI problems that have not resolved after you've used the first four steps for at least four

to six weeks. If they persist, revisit the first three steps with your provider or gastroenterologist to check if your child needs deeper diagnostics for gut inflammation or reflux, infectious disruptive gut microbes, or prescription medications that may alleviate symptoms. Some children need stronger or repeat rounds of antifungal medication to succeed with Step 2.

6. Consider heavy metals screening and treatment (chelation). Toxic loads of metals such as mercury or lead have been noted in children with autism to a degree that is higher than typical peers. These metals indefinitely impair digestion, immune function, cellular chemistry, and nerve function. Many children with autism have improved dramatically with chelation, which is a process that forces expulsion of these toxic metals from the body. It is a challenging process that requires a skilled provider's guidance. Children should be in the best possible nutrition status prior to chelation, and need monitoring during chelation for status of essential mineral nutrients.

7. Consider measures to reduce viral load or correct immune dysregulation. If all measures above have been tried for a year with little progress, it is time to check viral titers in your child. Many children with autism have been found to have extremely high antibody levels to some of the viruses they were vaccinated against. Treating this is effective in some cases.

WHEN, AND FOR HOW LONG

Plan to get your child through the first four steps in four to six weeks—a quick pace to accomplish a lot, but doable when you plan the needed changes in your kitchen ahead of time (see Chapter 6).

Choose a stretch of time when you can give this the attention it needs. Some families like to start during school breaks, when they don't have too many plans. Others prefer to start during school in order to get teacher feedback. In that case, it works best to keep the diet changes quiet at first. This will give you an opportunity to get completely unsolicited, unbiased feedback from teachers, friends, or family. It also means you avoid having to explain plans for a new diet to people who may or may not be supportive. Expect to notice some clear shifts in your child's abilities or behavior in this early phase. If you don't, keep going; there is more work to do. If your child has lived in a state of autism, chronic illness, allergy, asthma, sensory dysregulation, or ADHD for years, it will take time for all the layers that may have been physiologically challenged to right themselves. Plan to work with nutrition interventions indefinitely. This does not mean your household will be weighted down with unbearable diet restrictions for years to come. It may mean that you use some of these measures for many years, whether it ends up being a supplement or two, avoiding just one inflammatory food, or rotating measures throughout the months to boost immune function and focus.

WHEN TO GET HELP

Six to eight months is a very reasonable time frame in which to see dramatic changes with a special diet measure. If you haven't seen positive changes, something is missing from the intervention. Out of hundreds of children I have worked with on this, perhaps a dozen have shown no response. That is, their appetites remained rigid, bowel habits stayed the same, their developmental features did not shift. In these cases, deeper digging with specialists in chelation therapies, GI care, or immune therapies usually yields results. The sooner you move toward whatever other biological treatments may be helpful, the better, and your child will have the benefit of embarking on those in the best possible nutrition status, if the diet part has been executed well. If signs and symptoms of bowel trouble persist unchanged, or your child has shown no change in developmental signs, even though you've implemented an adequate diet—with new foods, the right supplements for your child, and supports for bowel symptoms (Steps 1 through 4)—for eight months, it's time to ask your provider network for more help.

As you implement diet measures, be aware of these signs and symptoms of inflammation from foods or malabsorption—they should be diminishing: Mixed irritable stools (hard pebbles with loose stool), exceptionally foul stool, a bowel movement less than once every two days, bloating, gas, frequent hiccups, loose or mucousy stool, or stools that are gold, green, black, or gray-white colored. Another important sign is pain: Children who are nonverbal will express GI pain with tantrums, aggressive or violent behavior, crying, pressing their stomachs on a flat surface (table, floor, pillows), pressing knees to chest, or sleeping with knees to chest. If you see these in your child, the first four steps are likely to help a great deal, if not eradicate this altogether. If you still see your child manifesting pain in this way, your child needs to see a GI specialist to rule out ulcers, esophagitis, persisting reflux, or infection with pathogenic bowel flora such as *Helicobacter pylori*, Clostridia, Candida, other disruptive bacteria, or parasites. Your specialist may recommend a drug such as Pentasa, which treats inflammation in the gut, or other measures to relieve symptoms. Singulair, a drug originally created for asthma, can relieve inflammation in the gut as well. In some children, Singulair has shown a side benefit of reducing anxiety. This supports my experience in practice that children with chronic inflammation from foods have more anxiety and more hypersensitivity to noise, light, and tactile input, and that avoiding inflammatory foods can improve these symptoms. For more about screening for foods that trigger inflammation in your child, see Chapter 3.

Some Nuts and Bolts About Child Nutrition: What You Need to Know to Succeed

For children, growth comes first. It is an irrefutable barometer of what is going on in a child's gut—a direct expression of what they eat and how well they absorb it. We all have a genetically programmed growth potential, and your child reaches it when diet and absorption are both adequate. Even if you think your child is growing well enough, address this piece first. This can tell you if your child needs more or less of any particular macronutrient, if he needs help absorbing a macronutrient, what foods might work best, or all three, without any lab testing. "Macronutrients" are calories (also referred to as energy), protein, fats/oils, and carbohydrates. While adults can get away with big deficits in any of those for a while, children simply can't. If your child is already operating under a deficit for any macronutrient, it needs to be identified and corrected at the start of special diet measures. Otherwise, you will not be able to tell which problems your child is manifesting due to an inadequate diet (the bottom layer), and which problems exist because of other treatable nutrition problems, such as inflammation from foods, inadequate digestion, intestinal candidiasis, cellular toxicity, and so on. When these higher layers are tested and treated first, as is often true in DAN or biomedical interventions, an inadequate diet can persist undetected. The result can be a powerfully negative impact on a child, and a derailment or stalling of your well-intended efforts with biomedical treatment.

"Micronutrients" is a fancy word for vitamins and minerals. Much of the biomedical movement's contribution has been in understanding the role of micronutrients in kids with autism spectrum disorders and its other diagnoses such as sensory integration disorder or ADHD. While this has made for some major breakthroughs for recovery and treatment, it falls second to the fact that children are growing and must have macronutrient needs met first. All else takes a backseat to this in any nutrition intervention for a child, and the only way to correct this first layer is with the right balance of appropriate macronutrients—that is, food.

CARBOHYDRATES: DO NOT BE AFRAID!

One of the most common blunders I encounter in children using special diets is that carbohydrates are overrestricted. This has been an overshoot of advice often heard to limit carbohydrate intake in order to control yeast overgrowth in the gut. It is true that yeast thrives when fed simple sugars (ever baked bread?), and that kids who have intestinal candidiasis (yeast infection in the intestine) need to avoid that. According to recent research, children with autism spectrum challenges frequently have intestinal candidiasis; when this infection is treated with anti-fungal agents, they improve dramatically. But it is also true that, just like yeast, children need carbohydrates to grow. Children need carbohydrates, period. They cannot grow well on Atkins-like food intakes, even when the total calories are adequate. Carbohydrates fuel weight gain; children need to gain weight, because they are growing. Adults are not growing. We can manage on a food intake that harshly restricts calories from carbohydrate while boosting protein and fat intake, but kids can't. It is a nonnegotiable reality of learning and development as well: By far, the brain's preferred energy source is glucose, which is derived from carbohydrate.

Carbohydrates fill an important role in the growing child. They are the primary fuel source, and as such, spare dietary proteins and fats for other important jobs only they can fill. Proteins are needed for tissue construction and functional molecule manufacture (hormones, neurotransmitters, enzymes, immunoglobulins, etc.). Fats are needed to make cell membranes work right, help us absorb certain nutrients, make up much of brain and nerve tissue, and are a component of many other structures and functional molecules. Children who must rely on dietary protein and fat for energy do not grow or function as well, and can end up overproducing toxic by-products of fat and protein catabolism such as ketones, urea, and ammonia. I have encountered many children in this situation who improve dramatically when appropriate carbohydrate foods are restored in their diets. Instead of withholding carbohydrates from your child's food intake, rotate antifungal medications or herbs into the routine, and supplement high-potency probiotics on a regular basis. More on how to use these is in Chapters 4 and 5.

Obviously, if your child has a body mass index that is nearing 30, or there are concerns for being overweight or obese, some strategizing needs to happen around limiting food intake and avoiding excess empty calories. Still, somewhere around half to two thirds of your child's food intake should be carbohydrate calories. Various strategies exist to ensure that these are healthful carbohydrates, which children on the spectrum are more inclined to eat once dietary opiate foods are replaced. More on that in Chapter 6.

OPTIMIZING FATS, PROTEIN, AND CARBOHYDRATES FOR YOUR CHILD

Children need healthy fats for normal brain and nerve growth, among other things. Do not restrict fats in your child's diet. Use healthy fats liberally, unless your child is above the 85th percentile for body mass index for age, that is, overweight. In that case, if calorie restriction is considered appropriate, you can still use healthful oils to about 25 percent of your child's total calorie intake, or somewhere between 40 and 50 grams per day for a school-age child (the exact number will depend on your child's weight, age, and percent ideal body weight). Do not omit them altogether. Healthy fats include omega-3 oils (supplements, fish, flax), avocado, safflower oil, olive oil, organic animal fats (meats, chicken, poultry, pork), organic eggs (especially with higher amounts of omega-3 fats in them), fresh oils from organic nuts or seeds, and even coconut oil. Coconut oil exists largely as medium chain triglycerides (MCT), which are easy to absorb—a bonus for children who have gut impairments, low output of digestive enzymes, or need more easily digested calories. It also contains fatty acids that have some antifungal properties, another bonus for kids on the spectrum, who often show overgrowth of fungal (yeast) species in the gut. Organic dairy fats are acceptable, too, if your child is able to tolerate dairy foods. While butter is omitted from casein-free diets (melt it and you'll see the protein solids in it appear as white stuff), organic clarified butter (ghee) is an expensive but rarified casein-free treat that can be used for special baking needs that demand the hardness and flavor of good butter. Melt that, and it looks like oil; at room temperature, it makes baked goods delicious and gives them perfect texture. Healthy fats, of course, exclude trans fats, hydrogenated fats, genetically modified or engineered oils such as canola oil, too many omega-6 oils such as soybean or corn oil, or rancid nut or seed oils, which can trigger oxidative damage in cells. And why organic? Because many agricultural chemicals and livestock hormones are lipophilic, that is, they like to situate themselves in fatty or oily places. To get the healthy fats without the risk of eating these other chemicals, look for reliable sources of organic foods.

Adding Therapeutic Oils

Oils and fats have the same calories per teaspoon, but differ vastly for functions in the body. Besides the fact that children absolutely need a certain percentage of calories from fats and oils, you will probably want to add certain oils as a therapeutic supplement. This has shown promise for children with autism, ADHD, learning disabilities, tactile hypersensitivity, inflammation, or mood concerns. For a full rationale from the nutritional biochemist's point of view, see the resources section. Here's the short explanation: Children with autism and ADHD are two groups noted to have abnormalities in fatty acid metabolism. These abnormalities have been linked to symptoms such as dyspraxia (poor gross motor coordination), auditory and visual processing disorders, aggression, mood swings, and dyslexia. Fatty acids that relate to these are typically poor in American diets. We tend to eat too few omega-3 fats and too many omega-6 fats, a ratio that has been linked to poor learning in rats: When fed a diet with too much 6 and not enough 3, they did really badly in that maze. Shifting this ratio so that more omega-3 fats are on board appears to positively impact these symptoms.

Phrases such as "omega-3," "omega-6," or "trans fats" refer to the chemical structure of the fatty acid. Fatty acids are long chain molecules with different configurations for where they hold hydrogen atoms. Hydrogenated fats are filled up with hydrogen molecules at every possible point, which makes them stiffer—too stiff. Great for a good piecrust, bad for your brain. Healthier fatty acids have some carbon atoms linked directly to other carbon atoms in the chain, without hydrogen in there. This makes for more fluidity in the whole molecule. Trans fats occur less often in nature and have a geometric configuration that makes them much harder to break or transform into other shapes or molecules in the body. They are thus bad at a major function of fatty acids, which is acting as a component of a cell wall. Cell walls need selective fluidity to let the right materials come and go in and out of the cell. Trans fats and hydrogenated fats make cell walls too stiff and dysfunctional. Preferable molecules for this job are omega-3 fatty acids, which make up somewhere around 8 to 10 percent of brain tissue and are a key component of myelin sheaths on nerve cells. Myelin is a material akin to insulation on electrical wiring in your house; it encapsulates the nerve fiber and permits smooth nerve impulse transmission. Research is active in how these fatty acids impact psychiatric disorders such as bipolar depression and schizophrenia, and other problems such as attention deficit disorder, hyperactivity, or aggression.

Signs that your child may need more of these fats are poor eye contact, night blindness, sensory dysregulation, tactile hypersensitivity, hostile or aggressive behavior, mood swings, skin rashes or dry flaky skin, or attention problems. While lab studies exist to refine exactly how you should best dose your child for supplemental oils, you can safely begin by giving 1 teaspoon of cod liver oil daily to a child over 40 pounds, and a half teaspoon daily to smaller children. Children who have struggled with frequent infections or who have just received a viral vaccination can use 1 teaspoon daily for the first two weeks, then go down to a half teaspoon daily. Generally, your young child's total intake of vitamin A, which is in cod liver oil along with these helpful fats, should not exceed 5000 IU per day on a long-term basis (more than three months). Check other supplements and fortified foods for the total amount your child gets daily. Signs of too much vitamin A, a nutrient we store rather than excrete, are bone pain (children may complain of pain in long bones, especially legs), hair loss, diminished appetite, or headache. Signs of needing more are photosensitivity (hates sunlight), lack of eye contact, stimming on fans, blinds, or lining up objects, frequent infection, night blindness, or dry scaly skin (this usually looks like crackle glaze skin or raised colorless/white dots on limbs).

Here are two examples of excellent results that I have witnessed in practice using fish oils:

- A boy age three with an autism diagnosis and poor eye contact was given a half teaspoon of cod liver oil for the first time. On the second day of using it, he sat at the breakfast table staring his mother down, right in the eye. According to the giddy phone message she left me about this, he appeared both dumbfounded and intrigued with this new ability, as though seeing his mother's face for the first time.

- A girl age five with ADHD and LD diagnoses who raged at clothing so badly that she tore all her clothes off in the car every morning on the way to school became able to remain calmly dressed after two weeks of 2.5 grams of eicosapentanoic acid (EPA) and 2 grams of docohexasanoic acid (DHA) daily, from fish oil. The battles about tags, socks, and seams ended.

Those are fast and dramatic changes. Most children begin a more gradual move toward better sensory regulation, behavior, attention, or eye contact after a few weeks. Fish oils should be used for four months before you review benefits. Depending on how long your child's diet supplied an upside-down ratio of omega-3 to omega-6 oils, it can take this long for these oils to be fully incorporated into cell membranes. Keep a journal if you can, as it is easy to dismiss slow shifts in the right direction; then compare your first entries to the last, months later. The vitamins A and D in cod liver oil (not present in other fish oils) also help immune function, and will help stave off winter colds, flu, and infection. Vitamin D at 2500 IU per day has been noted to shorten the course of upper respiratory infections in adults. In recent years, authorities have noted that most of us do not obtain enough vitamin D and may well need much more than previously thought. This nutrient is crucial for bone health, too.

Both EPA and DHA are omega-3 fatty acids, and they seem to have different merits. One researcher summed it up by saying "DHA is structure, EPA is function,"* referring to their roles in cell walls and in dopamine metabolism (dopamine is a neurotransmitter that relates to mood). If your child is prone to frequent infections, depression, and mood lability, cod liver oil may be a better choice, as it gives more EPA than DHA, along with immune-supporting A and D. You will want to give your child 2–3 grams of EPA daily in this scenario, which can be done with a teaspoon of cod liver oil and a teaspoon of Nordic Naturals Ultimate Omega Liquid, a concentrated version of fish oils that give over 800 milligram of EPA per half teaspoon. If your child's primary struggle is with dyslexia or attention problems, use fish oil that boosts DHA with a higher dose over EPA, anywhere from half a gram (500 milligrams) to a gram (1000 milligrams) per day.

To get enough EPA and DHA for a therapeutic effect, using gelcaps is harder than taking these oils in liquid form. High-quality oils

*Ralph Homan, University of Minnesota.

are now mostly odorless and flavored in ways that children accept, with citrus tones, allowing them to swallow spoonfuls in the higher doses needed for therapeutic effect (we use a scored medicine cup in our house). Keep fish oils refrigerated and out of bright light, and throw out old or rancid fish oils. If your child downright refuses a spoonful of oil, try mixing it in an ounce of lemonade or Sprite. While chewable gelcaps are a great idea for kids, your child would have to eat them by the dozen on a daily basis to get a relevant dose. These may be fine for children without specific mood, learning, or developmental concerns, but they are less suitable for proper dosing in the context of autism, ADHD, or learning disabilities. That said, if your child loves chewables, is willing to eat 10–15 DHA gelcaps per day, and you don't mind the cost, then stick with whatever works. If you don't notice the changes you're after, then you may want to pursue lab work to define exactly what fatty acid supplementation would work better.

How Much And What Types Of Protein Are Best For Your Child?

We've talked a little about carbohydrates and fats in children's diets. What about protein? Protein is not needed in terribly large quantities in a child's diet, but it does need to be of high value, be absorbed well, and it should not trigger inflammation or exogenous opiate compounds (see page 111 for an explanation of the Opiate Theory). Protein should usually make up anywhere from 12 to 18 percent of a child's total calorie intake. In terms of growth, well-absorbed protein in adequate quantity will generally permit expected progress on your child's height for age chart. If progress for weight is okay but a child starts to drop off that height for age channel on the growth chart, I will suspect protein malabsorption or low protein intake. This means that growth velocity for stature is slowing down, which it should not do unless your child is done or nearly done growing, for the most part. While all children experience growth in their own quirky fits and starts, the CDC's growth charts are based on large population data to help clinicians adjust for that. A child who continues in the same weight for age percentile while dropping off for height for age is eating adequate total calories, but is probably not eating or absorbing enough protein.

It is useful for children to have high-quality protein items regularly throughout the day, and especially in the morning. All that stuff about how breakfast matters is really, really true, especially for children, and it is well documented. Until a child has begun special diet treatments and has withdrawn dietary opiate sources, it will be exceedingly difficult to get them to accept protein sources other than their preferred wheat and dairy foods. It may also be difficult to get them to eat any protein in the morning at all, or anything at all. Before you try to change your child's eating patterns by simply presenting new foods, follow the sequence of steps outlined in this chapter. Very often, this will change the child's eating pattern itself, or at least make him more open to the changes you present. See Chapter 3 to learn how to incorporate lab findings into the steps described here. Once you have a good feel for whether your child's diet is adequate and how much food you are going to give daily, you can begin considering switching in new sources of protein to replace gluten, casein, or soy. Before you actually do, correcting bowel flora is the thing to do. Don't skip this step—optimizing bowel flora—explained in Chapter 3.

You may or may not need lab studies to define which types of protein will best suit your child. Some families like to start by withdrawing one protein—the one they most suspect is troublesome—and simply observing over a few weeks. Improvement is clear evidence that this protein was problematic. Continue with replacements of equal value for protein—if you pulled milk and cheese, put back the same amount of protein from healthy meats, eggs, or legumes your child will eat and can tolerate well. Chapter 3 discusses lab testing to look more deeply at this piece.

What Special Diets Do: Ketogenic, SCD, Body Ecology, Low-Oxalate, GFCF, and More

There are myriad special diet strategies now touted for children with special needs. If you use the steps in the order described in this chapter, knowing where to begin is easy, because the treatable nutrition problems will become plain in the assessment process. Since over-limiting of carbohydrates is the most common error I encounter in practice, I will start with carbohydrate restricting diets, and what they accomplish for special-needs children.

Carbohydrate restrictions for special-needs children are not new. One that has been applied for decades is the ketogenic diet, which has had some success in mitigating seizures. A ketogenic diet sharply restricts carbohydrate, gives most calories from fats, and gives more than the usual amount of protein. This forces the brain to use molecules called ketones, not glucose, for energy. Because this is such a dramatic departure from the ratios of macronutrients children need to grow and develop, this diet needs close medical supervision, and is usually begun in hospital. Why this can reduce seizure activity in about half to two-thirds of children who use it is unclear, but one possibility is that it starves out toxic bowel flora that rely on carbohydrate for energy. As you will see in the following section, disruptive strains of bowel flora (bacteria or yeast) can excrete toxins that are absorbed into the body and the brain. These toxins may disrupt brain chemistry, by engaging receptors for neurotransmitters or flooding them to a degree that seizures are triggered. And research has shown that children with autism can experience dramatic improvement with aggressive therapy for intestinal candidiasis or undesirable bowel flora like Clostridia.

I rarely place children with seizures on ketogenic diets, for two reasons: (1) This is a tool that staff at major medical centers are usually familiar with already. Parents can thus access an in-network (insurance-covered) team of providers there that can implement and monitor this challenging diet. It needs a team approach, with the neurologist on board, to coordinate dosing for medication if necessary. (2) I have found that children with seizures often improve dramatically with measures that correct overgrowth of yeast and disruptive bacteria in the gut, while key brain balance nutrients like magnesium, calcium, and pyridoxine are correctly replenished.

The benefits of a ketogenic diet for seizures may be related to some of the recent research findings in children with autism, who frequently also have seizures: They show intestinal candidiasis and florid overgrowth of disruptive bacteria more often than typical peers. One reason why this may be so, also confirmed with several studies to date, is that children with autism have pancreatic insufficiency and damaged villous tips more often than expected (these findings are only visible on endoscopy, a procedure done by a pediatric gastroenterologist that uses a scope to see inside the GI tract). If this is the case, they do not make enough enzymes to break down food, and the tiny structures meant to help further digest and absorb food do not work well either. Why would this be related to seizures? One possibility: Marginally digested meals get too far down the GI tract without being adequately digested or absorbed, where they end up feeding detrimental bowel bacteria, yeast, or parasites growing there. These microbes excrete their own by-products and toxins, which can circulate to the brain, impairing behavior, mood, or sensory modulation. The meal is finally expelled as poorly digested loose stool. Parents report stools that are frequent, explosive, gold or green, mucosy, or filled with undigested food. Carbohydrate restrictions can address this too-common accompaniment to autism, but can end up being too restrictive. Examples of carbohydrate-restricting diets popular in the autism community are the Specific Carbohydrate Diet and the Body Ecology Diet.

SCD and the Body Ecology Diet

Some families have had success with the Specific Carbohydrate Diet (SCD). This is a tool to restore gut health and normalize absorption, detailed in the book *Breaking the Vicious Cycle* by Elaine Gottschall. This diet aims to control overgrowth of Candida (yeast) and disruptive bacteria in the gut by only allowing carbohydrates called monosaccharides that are quick and easy to absorb in the upper small intestine. Monosaccharides that you may have heard of are sugars such as glucose, fructose, galactose, or ribose. They can't be broken down any further; they are as small as a sugar gets. The upper small intestine is the first section of your intestine that food enters when it leaves the stomach. Since yeast and other disruptive bowel flora tend to reside farther down the GI tract, the idea is to starve out these bugs by never letting the carbs they need reach them at all. Pivotal to the diet is using a home-made goat yogurt cultured with strains of healthful bacteria called *Streptococcus thermophilus* and *Lactobacillus*. These bacteria can help accelerate gut tissue recovery. The goat yogurt allowed on this diet supplies a good portion of carbohydrate calories for users of SCD, because the lactose in it is fermented into its smaller monosaccharide components, glucose and galactose. Otherwise, SCD relies mostly on certain fruits and vegetables for carbohydrates, though any with longer chain carbohydrates (disaccharides or polysaccharides) are also excluded. All grains are "illegal," including staples of gluten-free diets such as rice, tapioca, potato, or quinoa, as are all sweeteners derived from them, including cane sugar, corn syrup, maple syrup, and starches.

Like any specialized protocol, SCD has many devotees in the autism recovery community. I met Gottschall years ago and found her to be not only kind, delightful, and brilliant, but also full of wisdom about nutrition and children. But trouble with SCD usually happens for children with significant inflammation from all dairy protein, even goat dairy, and/or inflammation from other foods allowed on the diet.

Some children's bodies produce opiate-like compounds from dairy proteins, a problem about 80 percent of the time in people with autism (see page 111 for an explanation of the Opiate Theory). For those cases, the goat dairy is excluded. With so many foods disallowed to begin with on SCD, children who must avoid additional foods are not good candidates for this diet. Not only do they miss out on the key healing benefits of the goat yogurt piece, but they must replace the yogurt with other calorie sources. Since other carbohydrate sources permitted on SCD are often rejected by picky eaters, even the less restrictive, initial transition phase of this diet can be frustrating. I have observed that many parents give protein and fat sources to make up the difference. These include meats, fish, eggs, poultry, nuts, and nut butters. The plot thickens further here, because many children with autism spectrum issues are egg and nut intolerant, while others simply hate the texture of meat—leaving their choices even more limited on this diet. If this is your child, SCD is probably not for you. Because "legal" calories from other sources are so few, I have encountered children using SCD who eat five or six times their recommended daily level of protein—this would be something like 90–140 grams of protein per day for a small child. This is a protein intake that is more harmful than helpful. If your child has no sensitivities to the yogurt, eggs, or the many nuts relied upon for flours and baking, you may have success with this rigorous protocol. Support from experienced providers and families is advisable, as is monitoring of growth pattern and food intakes, to make sure both are as they should be.

Similar problems occur with other yeast control diets, such as the Body Ecology Diet. This diet uses certain combinations of foods eaten at certain times with supplemental enzymes and fermented foods to try to balance bowel flora. My concern with this diet is that, while full of potential for adults, it is too restricting for children. More than any other special diet for children, it also interferes with the normal social discourse of eating with family and peers, since users are expected to follow a strict schedule that dictates when enzymes and fermented foods are eaten relative to meals. Many carbohydrate sources are omitted. While I adopt a "whatever works" approach to helping children recover health and better functioning, this diet lost my nod of approval when I encountered a child in growth failure and protein calorie malnutrition while using it. Incredibly, the parents could not be convinced that this was more detrimental to the child's development than any benefit the diet might confer.

If you are using a diet like this and feel it is working well, check the growth parameters questions in this chapter, and tally the total calories your child eats daily. Compare what your child eats daily to the recommended total calorie levels. It will be clear whether or not your child's diet is adequate, using these tools. Even a small deficit in food intake will matter, if it persists for longer than one or two weeks. If a flattening of growth pattern emerges, or if the calories are lower than recommended, add more food to your child's day. If this can't be done within the framework of the diet, you need to flex that framework and add back any foods you know your child tolerates well, mostly as carbohydrate calories. Allow your child to eat as much of them as he likes, especially at first. Along with persisting negative changes in growth pattern, a sure sign that a diet is not adequate is if your child begins to succumb easily and frequently to colds and infections. Other signs are irritability, fatigue, sleepiness during the day and poor-quality sleep at night, and cravings for carb-dense foods.

Generally, appropriate carbohydrates for children on special diets include fruits, fruit smoothies, vegetables, starchy vegetables such as sweet potato, squashes, beets, green or wax beans, legumes if tolerated (black beans, chickpeas, kidney beans, cannellini beans), or gluten-free grains (and their flours) such as rice, buckwheat, tapioca, manioc, or quinoa. The SCD allowed-foods list is worth visiting (see www.SCDiet.org) even for non-SCD followers, since it illustrates that there may be more options than you thought for gluten-free foods or foods that are easy for your child to digest. Recipes are available at the SCD website as well. But strict yeast control diets can easily become inappropriate for children, because needs for growth and learning require a steady supply of glucose to the brain and cells. Instead of trying not to eat any food that might encourage yeast, I have found it to be much more effective to allow adequate, reasonable carbohydrate sources in children's diets, while rotating the yeast control tools mentioned above. That said, no one is advocating unlimited corn syrup and rice milk for kids on special diets. As inflammation in your child's gut calms down, and normal, healthy bowel flora are restored, digestion and absorption improve, thus permitting your child to tolerate a wider variety of foods.

LOW-OXALATE DIET

Equal mention should be given to the low-oxalate diet, which has come on the autism treatment scene more recently. This diet, which is not new in itself, aims to reduce the formation of irritating oxalate compounds in the body. Oxalates are crystalline molecules that can form kidney stones or gallstones, and adults with problems in that regard have used low-oxalate diets for decades. This diet was never intended for young children, and so far, most I meet who are using it are in calorie malnutrition. This does not mean it can't be a useful measure; it means that if you are using it, monitor your child's total food intake and make sure it is adequate. Or ask for help from your provider with monitoring adequacy of the diet. If growth has slowed, that is an irrefutable signal that you must give your child more food. Lethargy, irritability, frequent illness, and insomnia are typical signs of poor total calories as well. The low-oxalate diet is new to use as a special diet for autism, and many parents see improvements with it. Besides kidney stones or gallstones, oxalates can form highly irritating crystals in joint, gut, or virtually any tissue, including bone. These can trigger pain, irritability, and behavioral problems in children with autism, who have been shown to have highly elevated urinary oxalates more often than typical controls. This is probably due to having a leaky gut, that is, an intestine that is less selective than it should be about what it permits into circulation from foods and resident gut microbes. Oxalates that would normally be kept out of circulation may leak through, where they are very irritating. So, low-oxalate foods are permitted while high-oxalate foods are avoided. Foods omitted on this plan happen to be what are relied upon extensively in SCD: almonds, pecans, nut butters, carrots, and berries. Other high-oxalate foods are spinach, beets, chocolate, grapes, sesame seeds and tahini, soy products, and more. Urine tests exist to check for levels of oxalate, which can also be high in cases where intestinal candidiasis is very high. Treating intestinal candidiasis (that is, antifungal or antiyeast treatments) can in some cases bring down the load of oxalates, without having to avoid several more foods. A probiotic supplement called VSL3 has the ability to degrade oxalates in the intestine before they are absorbed, which offers another way to lower irritating oxalates for your child without overrestricting foods, total calories, or carbohydrates. This may help both by reducing intestinal permeability and by promoting manufacture of vitamin K, which can help direct calcium for deposition in the right places—such as bones and teeth—instead of the wrong places—such as soft tissue.

Making sure your child eats adequate total calories, protein, fats, and carbohydrates while remaining within the restriction is—as always—the key. When children show an initial excellent response to any restricted diet, but this improvement is not maintained weeks later, this often means that the diet has become inadequate. Revisit your child's total food intake and growth parameters, and add more allowable foods to boost intake. If this does not cause a return of those initial good results, talk to your provider about troubleshooting further. You may need to move to a different diet strategy if meeting your child's total food needs is too difficult within a given diet framework.

GFCF Diet

This is shorthand for the gluten-free, casein-free diet, popularized in the 1990s for children on the autism spectrum. Gluten and casein are the proteins in wheat (and some other grains) and in dairy products. In my early years working with this in practice, I quickly observed two things: One, this diet tended to become overly starchy and inadequate for protein for many children. Meats and eggs were not restricted, but many children would refuse to (or couldn't) eat them, thus they were left relying on rice milk or soy milk for protein. This created new problems. Two, many children had problems with inflammation from foods in addition to malabsorbing wheat and dairy proteins. This meant that a GFCF restriction alone was usually not enough to trigger dramatic benefit. The DAN/biomedical treatment community too soon realized that their initial somewhat blind enthusiasm for GFCF may have been shortsighted. It turned out that children on the spectrum had many more layers to treat than just removing wheat and dairy food. More detail on GFCF follows throughout the book. The diet basically withdraws all gluten and casein. This remains a reasonable initiation point, since these two proteins are the most frequent inflammatory trigger foods in autism, and the most frequently malabsorbed as opiate-like compounds. This is explained in more detail in Chapter 3. If you have tried this approach and saw no progress, take heart, as you may have just barely scratched the surface of treatable nutrition pieces for your child. As you will see throughout this book, there are many additional tools that can help you succeed.

Special Diet Strategies for Babies

If your baby has hard colic, lackluster growth, concerning developmental signs, persisting reflux, odd stools, or repeat infections, then something is awry for feeding and absorbing the baby's diet. If you are not breast-feeding, switch to casein hydrolysate choices like Nutramigen or Alimentum. If you are breast-feeding and the baby still has problems, consider switching off your milk. These are signs that it is not being normally absorbed, and as important as breast-feeding is, your baby may do better on a different feeding, with an addition of supplemental probiotics. If these do not adequately resolve symptoms, use a casein-free formula like Neocate. This gives the baby a completely allergen-free, safe diet; ask your pediatrician about it. If they aren't familiar with it, visit the Web for more information. Neocate has been used to relieve dermatitis and allergy in babies for many years, and can be successful. Soy formula may not be a worthwhile option, because many babies who struggle with casein also poorly tolerate soy protein, or acquire intolerance to it after a couple of weeks. If you've switched to soy formula and there are gradually worsening signs for constipation, bloating, reflux, or a slow return of eczema, then your baby is getting sensitized to soy protein. Best to go to Neocate in this case, and arrest all inflammation from feedings.

To further resolve colicky symptoms that won't quit, use baby probiotics with Bifido and Lactobacillus strains. Consider Diflucan for babies who have used antibiotics, who have shown thrush, when Mom had yeast infections in pregnancy, or who were delivered via C-section. Introduce solids slowly, and save gluten for later—perhaps after age twelve months, and try SCD-legal fruits and veggies at first, adding others as they appear to be tolerated. A child this age requires the bulk of calories to be carbohydrates with total calories at about 45 to 50 per pound per day (more than 100 calories per kilogram per day), so do not over-restrict. Carb sources like SCD goat yogurt; rice and rice cereal; taro, tapioca, and manioc flours or foods; sweet potato; winter squash; beets; or items like the gluten-free pumpkin bread in Chapter 6 are good starts.

Working Through the Nutrition Care Process for Autism, Step by Step

If you visit my website, www.NutritionCare.net, you will see the phrase "Nutrition Care Process for Autism" and the logo for NCPA. NCPA is an amalgam of biomedical and conventional clinical nutrition tools that has been reliably successful for me in practice. It is the proverbial phoenix that rose from the ashes of trials by fire I experienced as a parent and a health professional, working to provide nutrition supports for children in great need of them. These supports have only spotty availability in the provider landscape, and are rife with error when administered by inexperienced or unlicensed individuals. NCPA is my means of describing and standardizing this piece, so more health care providers and families know what it is and what to do. Ideally, any child with an autism diagnosis will be directed to a nutrition assessment early on, so they can access a successful nutrition care process.

Step 1: Assessing Baseline Nutrition Status

As mentioned earlier in this chapter, the first step in NCPA is checking your child's baseline nutrition status. This step is so pivotal to success for children using special diets, that I give it a lot of room in lectures, in practice, and here as well. Nutrition status in children can involve review of dozens of individual nutrients, but it first assesses growth and food intake. Worldwide, growth is accepted as the single most important parameter to judge a child's nutrition status. When a child's expected growth pattern is restored, she functions better, and of course, it means her intestines are working normally to absorb her diet. Monitoring growth patterns and food intakes gives immediate, concrete information about whether your child's special diet is adequate. It also sets the baseline for the whole intervention. If the diet isn't adequate, it isn't effective, because children with inadequate diets struggle cognitively, get sick more often, sleep less well, and suffer behavioral, learning, and functional deficits. If you have begun biomedical treatments with supplements, chelation, or special diets, chances are nobody assessed your child's growth status or food intake as closely as it could have been to really make the intervention pop. While I always put this at the front of the nutrition care process for a child, doing so is regarded as a bit dull, overly simple, or pedestrian by a lot of MD providers. Biochemistry is where all the action is, where the breakthrough papers get published. And everyone loves a magic bullet. Wouldn't it be great if it were true that all any child with autism ever needed was methylcobalamin shots, *et voilà!* While the work on methylcobalamin is breakthrough stuff, kids still need to eat diets that support energy balance for growth and cognition, eradicate inflammation, and eliminate toxicity issues.

Is Your Child Growing As Expected?

Three things will impair growth in children—and thus, learning, development, and functioning:

- Not enough food ("inadequate total calories" or "poor total energy intake")
- Not absorbing the food normally ("malabsorption")
- All of the above

Many children I encounter have all of the above. You can actually tell if your child is just a small kid, a little skinny, a little short, too heavy, on his expected growth pattern, or struggling to reach it. The following tips show you, or your clinician, how to accurately assess growth status. These are not new tools by any stretch—they are simply underused in our managed-care landscape today, leaving many children with growth issues to slip through the cracks. It takes some time to look at growth data adequately, and most routine pediatric visits don't allow for this.

If you think your child's growth is not as it should be, the special diet you choose will have to correct that, in order to make supplements, chelation, or other therapies more effective, and to remove confounding effects of a poor nutrition on concentration, focus, cognition, sleep, and mood. If you don't have your child's growth charts, you might ask your pediatrician for them, or you can visit the CDC's website and put "growth charts" in their search engine. Print out charts for your child (make sure it's the right one for age and sex), and plot the points. Many parents keep growth information in baby books. I often use these to plot growth charts for a child from birth, when parents don't have the actual charts. This illustrates the child's lifetime growth pattern. Your child should stick to his growth pattern, generally speaking, throughout his lifetime. There should not be unexplained or unrepaired big dips that persist beyond three or four months. This exercise detects fluctuations in your child's growth pattern that your pediatrician either did not notice or did not think were relevant. Even large and abrupt problems with growth come into my office without the child's pediatrician ever having raised an eyebrow, so don't assume you'd know about it by now if there were a problem. Likewise, don't assume that what may seem like an insignificant trend on a growth pattern is unimportant – it may yield some clues for you about how to make your child feel and function better.

RULES OF THUMB FOR GROWTH PROGRESS

Here are rules of thumb to check growth progress, many of which you can check without a growth chart. For body mass index, which is a way to check if weight is progressing well relative to height, you can visit the CDC's website and put "BMI" in their search engine, then click on "child and teen BMI calculator." This will give you your child's BMI and percentile BMI for age.

- Has the child's growth tracked along the same percentiles on his growth chart, give or take 10 percent, most his life? Big changes off an established growth pattern signal trouble.
- Did the child's growth mostly follow the trend visible at birth, or did it change dramatically? For example, if your baby weighed 8 pounds 10 ounces and measured 20 inches (healthy big kid!) but then straggled down the growth chart for weight and length in his first year, something was awry. The timing of this growth regression will yield clues to what your child did not absorb normally way back then, and whether it is still a problem.
- Has the child dropped channel and stayed there? An example of this would be if a child falls from the 75th percentile for height to the 25th, and doesn't rebound back toward the 75th. Dropping channel implies a negative shift in absorption, total food intake, or both.
- Is the child's body mass index (BMI) near or below 13, or the 10th percentile BMI for age? Is it above 25–30, or the 85th percentile BMI for age? Healthy body mass index means that weight and height are proportionate to each other. BMI values for children usually fall somewhere between 14 and 23, or in the middle third of the chart that tracks body mass index for age. The CDC regards a BMI for age as dangerously thin when it is below the 5th percentile. If it is hovering near the 10th, I am always curious why, and check a child's growth pattern over time to see if this is due to a downward trend, or if this is simply this child's normal pattern. No need to wait for a child to tumble all the way off the chart, and thus need to dig him out of an even deeper hole! The CDC likewise

regards a child as obese when the BMI value itself is above 30, or if BMI for age is above 95th percentile. A child whose BMI for age is above the 85th percentile is regarded as overweight and at risk for obesity by the CDC.

- Is the child's weight to height ratio near or below the 10th percentile for age? Is it above the 90th percentile for age? Ideally, weight to height ratio falls in the middle of the growth chart, right around the 50th percentile. The CDC's website has growth charts just for weight to height ratio. These are usually used in young children, up to age three or four. After that, use the growth chart for body mass index for age.

- Is the child at the ideal weight for his height? A child should be at or above 90 percent of his ideal weight for height. If it is lower, malnutrition has set in to a degree that can impair functioning, cognition, and infection fighting. Think of it this way: If a child's ideal weight is 40 pounds given his age and height, but he weighs only 30 pounds, then he is at only 75 percent of his ideal weight. This is approaching severe wasting, a dangerous place for a child to be. This degree of wasting is rare in the United States. However, in my own practice, I have encountered several children with autism and Asperger's syndrome hovering at 85 to 88 percent of ideal weight for height. Parents are usually astonished to see what a difference it makes to restore those very few extra pounds the child was meant to have, per his or her genetically determined growth potential. See the resources section to learn how to identify your child's percent ideal weight for height.

- Is the child reaching his expected stature for age? See "Resources and Further Reading" to find out how to check this, or visit my website at www.NutritionCare.net, and use the growth monitoring interface. Malnutrition usually affects weight first, then height. If your child is not as tall as expected for his age, then this signals entrenched malnutrition that needs correcting right away.

■ If the child is under three years old, has he grown less than 1.75 inches in the last year? This is slower than usual growth that needs professional assessment for causes. If your pediatrician already knows your child has a problem like this, ask for a referral to a dietitian for full nutrition assessment, or visit NutritionCare.net for consultation and more information.

■ If the child is under five years old, has she experienced a plateau in weight gain that lasted more than three months? If yes, it's time for professional consultation and support. Ask your pediatrician for a nutrition assessment referral or visit NutritionCare.net for more information.

■ If the child is older than five years, has there been a plateau in weight gain beyond six months? Again, ask for that referral or get professional guidance.

■ A nutrition problem will affect your child's weight first, then height, then head circumference last. This can tell you how long the problem has been present when you plot your child's growth pattern on his growth chart.

■ A problem with inflammation from food proteins—food allergy or food sensitivity—can impair growth, and may affect progress for stature while progress for weight remains the same. If severe enough, it will impact both weight and height.

Growth is the sum in this equation:

Adequate Diet + Normal Absorption = Growth

If any of these screening tools listed above highlighted a growth concern, your next step is to check the other parts of this equation, to see how they literally add up.

CHECKING YOUR CHILD'S FOOD INTAKES: COMPLETING STEP 1

There are no lab studies to assess growth or food intake. These are assessed by reviewing growth data and food intake data. Many children who enter my practice are already using special diets, and I nearly always find that their food intakes are inadequate or imbalanced to a degree that can impede developmental progress and/or growth. Lab tests that check organic acids, cellular energy markers, amino acids, and neurotransmitters—routinely used in the biomedical treatment model for children with autism—can be skewed by poor or imbalanced food intakes alone. If there is an underlying deficit for total calories, the right protein and carbohydrates, enough fats, or for absorption, giving your child supplements to redirect this biochemistry can be of little value. This is one reason why children have such highly varied responses to therapeutic dosing supplements or even psychiatric medications, which work better on a platform of a well-nourished child.

While overweight or obesity may top the list of child health problems for many pediatricians, being at less than optimal weight is a problem I encounter more often, in the population of special-needs children I meet. When children don't eat and/or absorb enough food, their growth slows down. This can happen very gradually, so that nobody even notices, but this can still make it hard for a child with special needs to master learning or developmental tasks by impairing cognition, focus, sleep, or behavior. If your child's weight for age percentile has steadily been dropping throughout his life (instead of staying roughly on the same percentile), he is either extremely physically active, is not eating enough total calories, or is not absorbing his diet effectively. Or all three! If a drop in the height for age channel occurs a while after the drop in weight for age began, you are looking at entrenched malnutrition. Fixing this will make your child feel better and function better.

First, make sure your child actually eats enough every day. Many children with sensory processing challenges or autism spectrum diagnoses do not, because they are picky eaters with objections to food texture variations, or they can't eat in cacophonous, noisy settings like school cafeterias. Or, kids with autism may eat plenty of starchy junk, but poor protein and no fruits and vegetables. Others eat enough but don't absorb it properly, and this can show up as growth problems as well as bowel signs, shiners at eyes, pallor, or frequent illnesses. Still others overeat because they seem addicted to wheat and dairy foods (more on that later). Either way, your child needs to get the right amount of food daily to best function. Parents of poor, picky eaters, take heart: This "behavior" can change when underlying triggers are corrected, so your child can start eating better, without a behavioral intervention.

Use these rules of thumb about children's food intakes to see if your child gets the right amount of food daily:

- Children need about 1000 calories per day, plus 100 calories for every year of age. For example: A two-year-old needs roughly 1200 calories every day. A seven-year-old needs about 1700 calories every day. If you'd like more detail, see the resources section for a chart showing calorie intake recommendations by age and weight. This rule of thumb applies only to children in normal growth status. That is, they are growing as expected. If a child is showing regression (too short, too skinny, too small overall), then a lot of extra calories are needed for catching up. Catch-up growth is fueled by some protein, but mostly by carbohydrates and fats.

- Children who do not get enough total calories show irritability, anxiety, lethargy, crying more easily, difficulty focusing/inattention, and/or insomnia. Children with the extra challenge of an autism spectrum disorder may also show more reactivity, oppositional behavior, behavioral rigidity, tantrums, intermittent mastery of skills, or behavioral disintegration when chronically underfed. One ten-year-old child in my caseload actually fell asleep and wet his pants every day at school; both problems vanished when he was given adequate total calories daily with some special strategies we created for him. Prior to this correction, these problems were regarded as behavioral and developmental for this boy, owing to his PDD-NOS diagnosis. This illustrates why it is not only pointless, but counterproductive, to medicate children for attention, focus, or anxiety problems without knowing first if food intake is right. Psychiatric medications cannot fix an inadequate diet. Some worsen the problem by diminishing a child's appetite and food intake all the more.

- Nonverbal children who do not get enough total calories may wake at night and cry, may have voracious seeking behavior for food (prying into the fridge or cabinets at all hours), or may show a peculiar grimaced countenance that seems more like a nervous tick than a purposeful expression. If you note these concerns, record your child's actual food intake and check if it is adequate. Some children with autism do not reliably sense hunger even when they are verbal, so in either case, you need to make sure they are getting adequate total calories.

- Children with growth regression or growth failure need a lot of extra calories for "catch-up growth." Examples of this are a body mass index that is near or below 13 or 14, a body mass index nearing the 10th percentile for age after a clear downward trend, being at 88 percent of ideal body weight or less, or unexplained drops in either weight or height channel on the growth chart. Whether extra calories are best supplied as protein, carbohydrate, or fat, and from which sources, depends on the child. If your child stacks up as too thin for her height, and her height is normal for her age, give more calories as healthy carbohydrates and fats/oils; you may not need to increase protein. If stature and weight are both lower than expected (little for age overall), your child may need more of all three (protein, carbohydrate, and fats/oils), or may need to switch to a new source of protein that is better tolerated. If you'd like help, visit NutritionCare.net for consultation and support.

- Children who weigh more than 40 pounds need a minimum of 25–30 grams of high-quality protein daily, or about a gram of protein for every two pounds of body weight, whichever is greater. For example, a 75-pound child needs about 35–40 grams of protein per day. Infants need less in total because they are smaller, but need more per pound. Unless your child is recovering from an entrenched growth lag, surgery, burns, or trauma such as a broken bone or major injury, more is not necessarily better: Too much protein may raise ammonia and urea levels in blood, places undue stress on liver and kidney, and has been associated with osteoporosis, kidney disease, obesity, and cancer. Eating more than 2 grams of protein per pound per day is too much on a regular basis for children.

If you see that your child needs more food, how do you get her to eat it, and what should she eat? The following chapters go into this in detail, and as you will see, success with this hinges on treating layers sequentially, so that your child's appetite can self-correct. Meanwhile, use growth and food intake data as often as you need, to keep your special diet intervention on track. It's typical for progress with special diets to stall out from time to time. This can mean that the child's needs have changed but the protocol didn't. Time to change the protocol, and the first thing to check is if it gives enough food from the right sources. The growth monitoring tricks and food diary will tell you that. Once your child is situated on a special diet protocol, revisit his food intakes and growth pattern at least every six months, either on your own or with your provider. You can also do this anytime the whole project seems to nose-dive. Doing this will give you fast feedback on whether the diet is adequate. Even the most seasoned biomedical and special diet moms goof this part up, and are surprised when I find that their child's diet has slipped into being inadequate for total calories, carbohydrates, fats, or protein. They are also surprised to see how simply adding back the right sources and amounts of food—not an obscure new supplement or lab test—recovers dramatic improvements for the child.

So, make sure growth and food intakes really look right. Prove it to yourself by recording a food diary and checking it against recommendations for your child's age and size, and by putting the new growth data on the growth chart. If all passes muster, it's on to deeper digging. This is where lab studies come in. When it comes to nutrition care for children, these pieces critically precede lab data, or at least coincide with lab data—which is why this chapter precedes discussion of lab studies, coming up in the next chapter.

Last but Not Least: Fix Your Child's Food Intake Before Tinkering with Supplements

Many parents ask, aren't supplements an easier place to start? Some also wonder whether proceeding with special diets in general is a good idea if a child responds to a supplement. The truth is, dosing individual supplements in the context of multiple unassessed, untreated nutrition or gut problems will probably tell you very little. If you see some positive shifts with a single item, that may mean that this is one nutrient to emphasize after your child is in sound status for growth and food intake. Or, it may mean nothing: Some of the quirky needs for high doses of individual nutrients disappear with replenishment and restoration of basic nutrition status. The NCPA sequence of steps presented here is what I have observed in practice over the years to work most reliably, and this sequence places supplementation (micronutrients) after restoration of a diet that is adequate for total energy, protein, fats, and carbs (macronutrients).

Using biomedical and special diet tools, it's common for parents to get too focused on the supplements, and overlook the food. Many parents hope to find a special supplement that works wonders, and forgo the work of a special diet. That may be possible for children with lesser behavior or learning diagnoses, but I have not found this to be realistic for children with autism. Children are growing, and everything falls in line behind that, in terms of their nutrition needs. You might say that these are more imperatives than needs in children. If the basics aren't met with an adequate diet, children simply do not function well, no matter how many supplements they eat, inject, rub on, or inhale. Sprinkling your child with supplements while she is eating an inadequate or inappropriate diet is a little like trying to lose weight by drinking diet soda while eating cheesecake and big burgers every day. You have to fix the food part, period. Supplements can't stop inflammation or toxins from the wrong foods, and can't fix growth deficits caused by imbalanced total food intakes.

Another helpful reminder is that any supplement can only work as well as your child's weakest nutritional piece. If your child has a chronically marginal intake of essential fats and oils, omega-3 fatty acids, or total calories, he can take methylcobalamin, glutathione, spironolactone, or alpha-lipoic acid all day, and it probably won't change that he is whiny, anxious, droopy, sleeps poorly, or hates socks on his feet or tags in his clothes. Those issues often relate to foods, not individual supplements. That said, at the right moment, those supplements can make an astounding difference—it's all in the timing and sequencing. I have encountered children on forty or more supplements a day. This is not sensible. Many of these children are not getting better. The basic nutrition status piece is usually overlooked in these cases. If a child needs that many supplements to get by, something is usually wrong with the diet, the child's absorption, or the child's cellular chemistry. Fix these, and a less-complex supplement regimen is usually beneficial. While supplementation is appropriate for all kids I encounter, I have never needed to recommend dozens per day for a successful outcome. More information follows in Chapter 3 about identifying supplements that may be helpful for your child.

THREE

Making Sense of Lab Tests

Defining What to Do for the "One in Six"

Two questions many parents have are (1) Do I need to do lab testing for my child in order to start a special diet? and (2) When do I do these tests? As discussed in Chapter 2, the answer to the first question is: not necessarily. When following Nutrition Care Process for Autism (NCPA) steps, the first part that needs attention is making sure your child's diet is adequate to support her expected growth pattern, sleep pattern, cognitive ability, and behavioral picture. This is corrected using growth data and food intake data, not lab testing. Once you know your child's growth status and you've identified his needs for total food intakes, then you can begin the process of elimination that prioritizes other nutrition problems. Two tools prioritize nutrition problems: One is called the Nutrition-Focused Physical Exam, which anyone can do. The other is lab testing.

The second question—when to do lab testing—can begin with

Step 2 in the nutrition care process. This choice is individually priori-
tized and is typically decided based on financial limitations, health
care coverage, and issues at hand for the child. Using the Nutrition-
Focused Physical Exam *first* can help cut costs and prioritize lab testing, since infants and children quickly manifest nutrition shortages in
clinical signs and symptoms. Because of this, I have often found this
tool to be as reliable or even more accurate than lab data for directing
treatment.

Nutrition-Focused Physical Exam

This is a great assessment tool that is underused in the biomedical and
conventional pediatrics communities. It can be done by virtually anyone. Once you know how much food your child needs, consider starting with this tool instead of costly lab panel packages that promise to
provide a total nutrition assessment, which they can't do for children
because they don't include growth data and food intake data. Between
growth data, food intake data, and a thorough check of signs and
symptoms, you may have enough information to get started with a special diet plan and a few supplements, without lab studies. After you
give your initial plan a few weeks, you can then use lab data to refine
what to do next. In any case, larger problems made evident using this
Nutrition-Focused Physical Exam will need to be fixed before the finer
details found only with lab testing later on.

SIGN/SYMPTOM	RULE OUT/ASSESS
Low weight for stature	Chronic low total calories
	Diabetes
	Malabsorption of carbohydrate calories
	IgG food antibody responses
	Sensory challenges when eating

SIGN/SYMPTOM	RULE OUT/ASSESS
Height for age dropping channel	Chronic low total protein Protein malabsorption Gluten intolerance (antigliadin IgG) Diffuse inflammation from foods (IgG and IgE)
Decreased subcutaneous tissue	Chronic low total calories
Low muscle tone	Mitochondrial disorder Review vitamin/minerals status Heavy metals status Diabetes
Muscle wasting, weakness	Diabetes Protein, calorie intake, and absorption Mitochondrial disorders Cellular toxicity (heavy metals) Vitamin D, thiamin
Painful calf muscles	Thiamin, selenium status
Tetany	Calcium, magnesium status
Loss of reflexes, foot drop, wrist drop, numbness, tingling, heightened sensitivity	Thiamin
Loss of vibratory or position sense (vestibular sense)	Vitamin B12 Malabsorption/intrinsic factor Methylation
Dementia, disorientation	Niacin
Bloated abdomen, reflux	IgG food antibody responses Gut dysbiosis
Hiccups, wet frequent stool, gold stool, mucousy stool	Gut dysbiosis Pancreatic or gut enzyme insufficiency Inflammation from foods Inflammation from disruptive bowel flora
Constipation	Elevated dietary opiates Mostly wheat and dairy diet Disruptive bowel flora, Candida overgrowth
Stool incontinence	Inflammation from foods, disruptive bowel flora Elevated dietary opiates, Candida overgrowth
Poor appetite	Chronic low calories and protein Low zinc Marginal iron status

SIGN/SYMPTOM	RULE OUT/ASSESS
	Food antibody responses (IgG)
	Excess vitamin A dose (>5000 IU/day x 2 mos)
Rigid, voracious appetite	"Opiates" from casein, gluten
	Intestinal Candida overgrowth
	Low minerals, especially zinc and chromium
Salt craving	Adrenal fatigue, mineral deficiencies
Pica	Mineral imbalance or deficiencies (zinc, iron)
	Toxic levels of lead, mercury
Pallor	Low folate, iron, B12, B6, vitamin C
	Inflammation from foods
	Low protein intake
Follicular hyperkeratosis (raised white bumps) Dry eyes, mouth, or skin	Low vitamin A or essential fatty acids
Flaking dermatitis	Check for adequate protein, calories, niacin, riboflavin, zinc, essential fats
Easy bruising	Vitamin C, K, and EFAs; poor bowel flora
Persisting wounds	Low vitamin C, zinc, or protein
	Poor blood sugar control
Hyperpigmentation	Low B12, niacin, or folic acid; adrenal fatigue
Photophobia, conjunctival inflammation	Low vitamin A, riboflavin; rule out infection
Spooning nails Ridged nails White dots on nails	Low protein, low zinc, low iron*
Cracked peeling nails Frequent infection Bloated abdomen w/soft musculature Thin, dull, easily plucked or brittle hair Low stature for weight or age	Poor protein status
Redness at tips of ears Flush redness on one cheek Irritability with food dyes/pigments	Inadequate sulfation
Hard tender lumps at back of head	Excess vitamin A
Headache	Excess thiamin

*Serum iron may be low and total iron-binding capacity (TIBC) may be elevated.

SIGN/SYMPTOM	RULE OUT/ASSESS
Frequent, painful urination	High oxalates, low vitamin K, intestinal or uinrary tract candidiasis, urinary tract infection
Delayed sexual maturation	Poor zinc status; excess vitamin A or D Inadequate total calories, protein, fats
Skull flattened, prominent frontal bones, delayed skull suture fusion Knock knee, bow leg, beads on ribs	Low vitamin D, low vitamin C
Dull soft cornea, Bitot's spots (eyes) Night blindness	Low vitamin A
Burning, itching eyes Photophobia	Low riboflavin (check for low RBC glutathione reductase)
Redness/fissuring at corners of eyes	Low riboflavin, niacin
Pale membranes at eyes Redness at belly button Easily fatigued	Iron status, protein intake
Fissures, redness at corners of lips	Low riboflavin, B6; excess vitamin A
Magenta tongue	Low riboflavin
Pale tongue	Poor iron status
Red, swollen, raw tongue	Low folic acid, niacin, or B12
Spongy, receding, bleeding gums	Low vitamin C
Defective tooth enamel pitted/discolored enamel	Low vitamin A, C, D, calcium, or phosphorus malabsorption; excess fluoride or antibiotics
Arrhythmia, palpitations, rapid pulse	Excess niacin, potassium, magnesium Low magnesium, potassium, thiamin Excess lactate (lactic acidosis)
Seizures/convulsions	Low B6, thiamin, vitamin D, calcium, magnesium Rule out excitotoxins (glutamate, aspartate, MSG, Nutrasweet) or NMDA receptor dysfunction Rule out florid intestinal candidiasis Rule out lactic acidosis Rule out opiate polypeptides

Once you've perused this list of signs and symptoms, you will probably be thinking about supplements to add. See Chapter 5 for details on how to proceed—you won't want to quickly begin high doses or several items together. You can also see a list of vitamins and minerals (micronutrients) relative to signs and symptoms in Chapter 5, then make a list of the problems you note in your child. If you are working with a provider on the biomedical piece, be sure to share your findings with him, and discuss his ideas on supplementation.

It's after you've used some corrective measures—those that you found by checking growth, food intakes, and signs and symptoms—that you might proceed to lab studies. This is not necessarily the right or only way to work through a special diet program, but it is the most methodical, conservative, and possibly the least expensive. If you like, you can dive in with lab studies up front—but as has been pointed out already, this won't fix foundation problems with growth and food intakes that usually exist in special-needs children, problems that will impede your efforts with supplements and toxicity treatments later on.

If You Are Ready for Lab Studies, Where Do You Begin?

Now that one in six U.S. children is affected by some type of learning or developmental disability, an industry has popped up around this in the last decade. It is the business of using lab studies to gauge what might be going on with your kid. This industry provides direct parent access to lab tests for children affected by autism spectrum disorders, sensory integration, ADHD, ADD, learning disabilities, mood disorders, and other challenges. Parents can order tests directly off the Internet, and get a phone consultation on results with a staff person at the lab. No face-to-face time with a doctor happens. No one meets your child, or you. There is a dizzying array of choices. The outcomes usually suggest therapeutic supplements. Every website and every autism conference vendor booth touts its product and approach as the top priority for an affected child's well-being. Besides these confusing choices, providers in the biomedical community often insist on their own preferences for unconventional lab tests to define toxicity, inflammation, or metabolic problems in these children. Frequently, these tests are denied by health insurers, so parents pay out of pocket for many of them. This is a new and blurry zone of medical care that—like every part of the "one in six" conundrum—has both passionate supporters and fervent detractors.

As parents struggle to help their children behave, learn, socialize, and function better, they are looking for whatever works. The problem, and the reason why the lab test industry is blooming, is that there is no one place to go where a provider can piece this puzzle together. For children with challenges as deep as autism, anxiety, or intractable ADHD, care is often splintered across many disciplines. Neurologists, developmental pediatricians, metabolic disorders specialists, therapists of all sorts, and gastroenterologists might be in the mix. That gets expensive, and confusing. Parents are eager for a way to have some control over this circus. They also crave some action on the situation, while they wait through the agonizing months it often takes to see a specialist. Direct-access lab studies fill the gap for many families. For better or worse, parents have become partners in this process and need to know as much about it as possible, in order to assure better care for their children with special needs.

As parents turn to their battery of specialists, they often engage psychiatrists to prescribe medications for attention, mood, focus, anxiety, or behavior problems. These can work well alongside nutrition tools. It is helpful to remember that while psychiatrists know a lot about medications, they do not typically study nutritional biochemistry. For example: When one child in my caseload was being reviewed for anxiety medication, I asked the psychiatrist if tryptophan supplements (such as 5-hydroxy-tryptophan) should be avoided with this medicine, since the family was interested in both. His response was "What's tryptophan again?" That gave me quite a pause, because

I assumed that if any MD provider would remember what tryptophan is, it would be a psychiatrist. Tryptophan is an amino acid precursor of serotonin that is in foods and popular as a supplement for depression. Children with autism have higher amounts of serotonin in their blood than typical children, indicating that it may not be taken up into nerve cells normally. Mixing tryptophan with selective serotonin reuptake inhibitors (SSRIs) may escalate anxiety, activate the behaviors you are trying to quell, or even trigger a potentially fatal reaction. Luckily, the family was forthright with lots of questions, which meant that the child was given a safe protocol. Had they used supplements without the provider team's knowledge, things could have gone very differently.

What should parents do? Whether you are considering a lab test you've never heard of, or a medication you don't know about, the key is simple: *Ask lots of questions.* There are no dumb questions. How psychiatric medications actually work is often not well understood, which is why prescribing them can be a semi-informed roulette. Some urine tests offer profiles of neurotransmitters and their metabolites, ostensibly to predict which supplements or medications might be effective. But these still can't reliably indicate what is going on in the brain, or in synapses between nerves, where chemicals such as serotonin need a certain balance to work properly. How they work also has a deep overlap with nutritional biochemistry, and this is a yet-to-be-studied interface. Pharmaceutical companies are just beginning to market blends of drugs with supplements or herbs that enhance effects of the drug. Certain herbs and supplements, in countless combinations, can be very effective also, without drugs and with fewer side effects. Individuals vary so greatly for their own nutritional biochemistry that it will probably be a long time before there are reliable lab tests to predict which psychiatric medications might work well for whom. There are some sixty or so known neurotransmitters, all of which flux, wax, and wane day and night in different ways for everybody. There are more receptors for serotonin in the intestine than in the brain, and serotonin is produced in both places—in fact, as much as 90 percent of the serotonin in your body is in your GI tract. If your child's bowel is diseased, leaky, inflamed, or full of pathogenic flora, how does this affect serotonin chemistry, or how might an SSRI be tolerated?

It might seem wise to ask a gastroenterologist, who, after all, knows about the stomach, digestive organs, enzymes, hormones, and intestines every way to Sunday. The imbalanced bowel flora common in children with autism are capable of affecting the brain, when their toxic by-products are not safely detoxified by the liver. The toxins end up in general circulation, and in the brain, where they affect behavior, mood, cognition, or more. This is probably why antifungal medications such as Diflucan can trigger benefits for children with "one-in-six" issues— studies have demonstrated that children with autism frequently have intestinal yeast overgrowth. Clostridia overgrowth, a bacterial infection that triggers diarrhea, is found more often than normal in children with autism, too. Treating Clostridia with antibiotics improves bowel function and lessens autism features as well (but problems return once the medicine is stopped). Though a gastroenterologist may be willing to work with this information, he may not know much of anything about psychiatric medications or herbs that enhance serotonin, not to mention the other few dozen neurotransmitters that regulate focus, sleep, panic, calmness, happiness, alertness, aggression, and so forth. It's easy to see why this gets overwhelmingly complex very fast, and why the traditional medical model of parsing out body parts to different specialists can fall short for yielding answers. It also sheds understanding on why parents often turn to the Internet to buy lab studies, as they search for a clue or breakthrough to help their child.

Starting with the basics and moving methodically forward is one way families and providers can keep their heads from spinning. A process-of-elimination approach to lab studies can help refine treatment choices. This chapter will explain some of the tests commonly used, and some will no doubt be omitted here—but generally, if you are looking for nutrition or biomedical enhancements for your child's functioning, the tests mentioned in this chapter are what you are likely to run into. Though all providers have their preferences, I have the most success when lab testing for children with special needs such as autism, Asperger's, ADHD, or other learning, behavior, or mood disorders by using this order:

- Review of bowel flora (stool culture and/or urine screen for signature chemicals of toxic bowel flora)
- Food allergy or intolerance (ELISA IgG, antigliadin IgG; rarely, IgE testing or celiac screen)
- Toxicity (urine organic acid test ["OAT"], urine porphyrins, or oral challenge for heavy metals)

All of the tests described in this chapter are secondary to the *baseline nutrition assessment* discussed in the previous chapter, since any deficit for growth or food intake will impede and confound everything else in the child.

First, What to Avoid

For any lab testing suggested for your child, avoid tests that have no immediate impact on the care plan. It's appropriate for you to know the purpose of any lab test you buy, and what it means for treatment. For example, if your provider wants to check your child's homocysteine level, he should have a compelling reason why. Homocysteine levels may be repaired by chelation therapies or certain supplements. Recent research illustrates that homocysteine is a key molecule in autism spectrum disorders, but this new information has a long way to go before it trickles down into a standard of care that health insurers are willing to pay for. You may not get that covered on insurance, depending on who is ordering the lab work and how it is coded. Your question then becomes, exactly what treatment would be triggered by a finding of elevated or depleted homocysteine? If your child is extremely anxious and unable to tolerate the blood draw, or if your finances don't permit the lab work, ask your provider if there are other ways to get information about transsulfuration and methylation. These are the critical metabolic pathways for attention, detoxification, and cognition that use homocysteine to keep them humming. Important findings have emerged to explain how these pathways are barely functioning in children with autism spectrum diagnoses or ADHD.

Assessing methylation and transsulfuration pathways ideally uses blood work, but many nutrition-related problems in children can be ascertained with a nutrition-focused physical exam and by reviewing food intake and supplementation data. Through these tools, you can get a thumbnail sketch of whether treatment for this piece is indicated. Children with autism consistently show depressed homocysteine levels, which means that they are likely struggling under a toxic burden and oxidative stress to such a degree that behavior, cognition, attention, or language is impaired. Clinical features for impairment in these pathways may include reddened ear tips, one cheek red and the other pale, difficulty with phenolic foods or additives, or poor tolerance for ordinary doses of medications. There may be other more targeted lab values besides homocysteine level that can define the functionality of these pathways. Some providers are willing to begin treatment to correct this without lab studies. Discuss what best suits your comfort level and budget ahead of time. Treatment usually includes a sequential replenishment of the nutrients these pathways need: tri-methylglycine (aka "betaine"), folinic acid (not folic acid), and injectable or inhaled (nasal spray) methylcobalamin, all of which have excellent safety records. Oral methylcobalamin, which is the methylated form of vitamin B12, is not very effective in this treatment; cyanocobalamin, which is the form of B12 in most typical supplements, is not effective at all. Be sure your provider can satisfy your questions about treating an advanced piece like this, before you begin. Again, though some providers disagree, I favor stabilizing a child's growth and food intake before any toxicity treatment measures are introduced. For those who like to go directly to the source and don't mind academic, peer-reviewed articles for reading material, a list of research articles on this topic is in the resources section.

CLARIFY LAB FEES BEFORE YOU START

One practice I'd rather see parents avoid is being obligated to purchase lab test kits from providers and pay up front for all lab studies. Here's how it works: In the conventional care universe, parents rarely see a lab test kit or take one home. Blood, urine, or stool samples are usually collected at the clinic site and processed there or handled for you if they need to go elsewhere for processing. Billing to insurance is initiated for you by the provider's staff and you are not asked to pay at that moment. In the biomedical treatment universe, few providers have labs or an army of administrative staff on-site. They typically use tests that are unusual and unavailable locally. Lab test kits are usually given to providers for free by the labs, and providers then sell them to you, the patient. Blood may be drawn on-site or you may be sent to another facility for a blood draw, but the sample is processed somewhere else. For urine and stool samples, you may be given a kit to carry home, where you collect the sample and forward it to the lab for processing, via the packaging and FedEx materials included. Besides not having lab facilities to evaluate samples on-site, biomedical providers may be using lab resources in another state that specialize in what they are looking for.

That's fine enough if the test is warranted—more on that in a moment. But when a provider sells you a lab test kit, and doesn't give it to you for free, you are paying ahead of time for the lab work (which is done by the lab, not the provider), and paying a profit to the provider for simply handing you a lab kit that he got for free. The provider is then billed by the lab later on, when your sample has been processed, but at a discounted rate. Families of special-needs children have enough financial struggle, and this is one place where I believe providers should not be taking a cut. The provider in this scenario is essentially skimming an extra fifty bucks or more for every test he orders, just because he can. When it comes time to interpret the findings, he is probably going to charge you for the consultation anyway. If you are planning to work with a provider in the biomedical community, clarify exactly where fees apply ahead of time. Ask if the provider discount for lab fees is passed to patients—it can be, at the provider's discretion. Unless the provider is processing insurance claims for you—a time-consuming task that requires extra staffing—then there is little reason to charge you the extra fee. If you must buy lab kits up front, ask if consult time to interpret the findings is included with the purchase. Providers need to cover their costs and time, and their expertise is valuable, but reasonable fees should still apply. Ask your providers how they approach this. In my own practice, where my license permits me to authorize labs relating to nutrition care, I give kits to families, and let them decide how to pay. I am out of that loop and take no cut off that. Many labs will work with parents on this, and will either submit directly to insurance for you, or will offer a lower price to those able to pay early.

Prepackaged Panels and What They Can't Do

Combination "nutrition profile" panels have become popular with some providers in the biomedical treatment community as a matter of course for every new patient. I am wary of providers who insist on a battery of lab studies before they ever see your child, as a point-of-entry requirement for their practices. This is an effort to streamline the process of assessing children, especially those on the autism spectrum, who as a group tend to show many of the same biochemistry problems over and over. While I can appreciate the desire to simplify this process, this is an expensive way of doing it much of the time, and thus available only to families who can put up the few thousand dollars out of pocket that it can cost. Explore ahead of time if this can be submitted to insurance for you, and what the odds for coverage are. Find out how your provider plans to code it. Any nutritional therapies coded under a developmental, psychiatric, or behavioral diagnosis code will be refused by insurance. Your provider should choose the nutrition or metabolic diagnosis codes that apply to the initial findings, which is another reason why he ought to meet your child before ordering lab work—he can't code a lab order without knowing first what diagnosis codes apply to the order, and it should not be a code for "autism."

Besides expense, another drawback is that because they are a one-size-fits-all approach, lab packages usually have at least some testing in them that is downright useless—rarely does every test in it apply to every child. Why pay for it? If your provider favors these tools, ask exactly what all the lab findings will trigger for treatment. Perhaps he would be willing to work with you in stages to help accommodate your budget. This can make good clinical sense, too, since it can be challenging to treat more than two or three things at once in a child.

In my practice, I have not found a particular package of tests that answers all the nutrition questions I have when I meet a child for the first time. Counter to what they imply, prepackaged "nutrition profile" lab studies do not provide a complete nutrition assessment for a child. No lab test can, because nutrition assessment for children has five components, usually evaluated in this order when professional standards of nutrition practice are followed:

1. Anthropometric measurements (current height, weight, body mass index, and parameters to assess growth rate and status, like percent ideal body weight or height-age equivalent) and review of growth history.
2. Quantify food intake and review activity level (exactly how much and what does the child eat, and what is the child's physical activity level/capability).

3. Review of clinical signs and symptoms with a Nutrition-Focused Physical Exam.
4. Review of the child's medical history, including social and family contexts, housing, access to needed measures, and health history.
5. Biochemical data, medical tests, procedures, or lab data.

A biochemistry panel in itself is never a total assessment of a child's nutrition status, and it alone does not yield enough information to make a nutrition care plan, because it doesn't tell you how much food the child needs daily or what growth status is. Growth status and food intake are the foundation pieces to review for children, before lab studies are chosen. This is simply good practice, and it has also been the standard of care for child nutrition for decades. Lab data can fill in missing pieces, but assessing growth and food intakes first will answer many questions before blood, stool, or urine samples are collected. Medical history and family or social contexts are important, too, because at the end of the day, parents need to know what to make for dinner for their household, not what supplements to give one child in the house. Adding standards of child nutrition assessment, instead of using lab data by itself, makes biomedical treatment tools and special diets safer and more effective. Though individual assessment like this may take more time, it ferrets out which tests are truly useful in your child's case, and which ones are probably not going to yield any workable results.

BEFORE A DROP OF BLOOD IS DRAWN, ALWAYS START WITH SIGNS AND SYMPTOMS

This is yet another reason why a good provider will want to meet you or your child *before* ordering lab studies. Nutrition problems are reliably evident in a child's clinical presentation. This can help streamline lab work, and it can reduce the number of tests you need to do.

Identify and Treat Problems with Gut Bacteria: Why and How

Once you have used growth and food intake assessment tools to get a feel for how much food your child needs in a day, you are ready for the next piece, Step 2 of NCPA: balancing gut bacteria (also called bowel flora) for optimal digestion and absorption. It is the second step in a good nutrition care process for children with special needs, because it is crucial to balance bowel flora as much as possible before, or very early in, the process of using special diets or supplements. You may or may not need a lab test to balance bowel flora. Tables later in the chapter identify signs specific to imbalanced bowel flora, to help you prioritize when to use a lab test for this piece. But first, it's useful to know how pivotal healthy bowel flora may be in your child's improvement.

Bowel flora are all the microbes that inhabit the gut. Several species of bacteria, parasites, worms, viruses, and yeast, weighing somewhere around three pounds in an average adult and virtually impossible to count (estimates run into the hundreds of trillions of cells), can reside in the human gut. Identifying all the species would be literally impossible for any individual, let alone a clinical trial group or a population study group, but there are undoubtedly hundreds and perhaps even thousands of species. Bowel flora eat what you eat. Here's a useful analogy: No gardener throws a nutrient-rich compost tea on a weed patch. Gardeners yank or kill the weeds first, perhaps mulch the weed-prone areas, making space for the plants they'd like to grow. *Then* they fertilize. Fertilizing ahead of weeding will give you more weeds, which usually end up crowding out the desirable plants. This is a little like bowel flora. There are important and beneficial strains you want to keep, and detrimental or downright pathogenic strains you need to purge. Once this is balanced, you can add nutrients without losing them to hungry gut bugs that undermine infection fighting, digestion, detoxification, or absorption. Even though gut flora profoundly influence digestion, absorption, and drug metabolism, this is little-studied area of medicine. It is a bit of a hot potato, tossed between medical specialties at the moment. Should it fall under microbiology, gastroenterology, nutritional biochemistry, functional medicine, toxicity, or all of the above? There is no clear answer, and there is a lot we don't know about human intestinal flora.

What we do know is that the first two years of life are a critical window for acquiring the necessary helpful bacteria in a baby's intestine. The right balance will help a baby digest food normally and will help fight infection. The wrong balance can trigger intestinal permeability ("leaky gut" syndrome), food allergies or intolerances, constipation, irritable stools, or frequent illness, and can interfere with growth. Digestion of first feedings in the newborn's sterile gut are meant to be aided by that first exposure to bacteria in the birth canal, and at Mom's breast. One gastroenterologist I have met called this mouthful at birth the "vaginal gulp" and regarded it as an important first imprint for the baby's immune system. So far, bacteria known to be beneficial at this stage are Bifido bacteria and some strains of Lactobacillus. Healthy immune response to viruses and unwanted bacteria are supported by beneficial flora in the human gut, which receives ongoing exposures via swallowing. Some beneficial bacteria actually produce natural antibiotics that kill other detrimental species.

Both these "skills"—that is, normal digestion of breast milk or formula, and effective immune response to pathogens entering by mouth and swallowing—are essential to a baby's survival, growth, and development. When the process of building this digest-and-defend system in the baby's gut is interrupted, how does the baby's intestine evolve, for structure and function? How does this affect growth and development? These are big questions for special-needs children, who often show problems with intestinal flora and gut function.

While this is wide open for study, the answer seems to depend on the severity and timing of the interruption in this process. Antibiotics disrupt normal bowel flora. Children are now routinely given antibiotics, sometimes repeatedly, well before age two. For those babies with very early antibiotic exposures, including through Mom's breast milk if Mom is on antibiotics, no one can say at this point what this means for the immature immune system, especially when vaccines (which impart even more "data" to the immune system) are given around the same time. Antibiotics kill bacteria; when they are needed to kill a pathogen in the body, the collateral damage is that they kill beneficial intestinal flora as well. This lowers the protective effects of beneficial bowel flora at a time when the baby most needs it. This may even wholly eliminate the beneficial flora if the baby has not had enough time to develop mature, healthy bacteria colonies in the intestine. This is why adults can use yogurt or Lactobacillus supplements after antibiotics, but babies may need this even more—to protect the normal development of gut function, to prevent food allergies and sensitivities as they introduce solid foods, and to permit optimum absorption of food.

After assessing so many young children with histories of multiple, early antibiotics, I have wondered if this affects development and immune function much more than we know. When antibiotics are given very early, say in the first weeks of life, the baby's immune system is so immature that it may have trouble recovering that "digest and defend" sequence in the gut. An error message may be given to the baby's new immune system to teach it to regard disruptive flora as normal. I say this since I have met many children with autism who are utterly unable to retain normal bowel flora, no matter what medications, diets, probiotics, or supplements they use; the bad stuff won't quit, and just keeps growing back. Signs of struggle for bowel flora during infancy can include poorly tolerated feedings from the start, vomiting, hard colic, mucousy stool, explosive stool, heavy cradle cap or eczema, gas, difficulty feeding, persistent diaper rash, thrush, pulling off the breast and crying, or spitting up that is too frequent and too hearty.

The most altered growth and development I have encountered in practice is in infants and young toddlers who have had been exposed to antibiotics early and often. In a few cases, this appears to have created food intolerance, malabsorption, repeat illness, and reflux so severe that a gastrotomy tube is required. This is a tube surgically inserted directly into the stomach to deliver feedings, because the baby is unable to eat enough by mouth to survive. I have wondered if extreme outcomes like this could be lessened or even prevented by building in healthy bowel flora supports from day one. Disruptive bowel flora is like a greedy middleman: Everything your child eats, including supplements, has to pass through this stuff, and just like a middleman, the flora takes its cut, by consuming vitamins, minerals, some amino acids, and carbohydrates that your child needs. Worse, the flora leaves its own garbage behind after its picnic, which your child absorbs. Get rid of it, and the sooner, the better. In children with autism, bowel flora that are only supposed to reside in the colon, or the back end of the GI tract so to speak, have also been found in the small intestine, closer to the stomach. They are not supposed to be there, and if they are, they will interfere with digestion and absorption.

Using Probiotic Supplements

How to choose and dose supplemental healthy flora, or probiotics, is a burgeoning area of practice. Like any medicine, supplement, or medical food, not all probiotics are created equal—there are strains of good bacteria that will work well for some children in some circumstances, but badly for others at other times. Probiotics are widely available online and in stores. Some makers of probiotics stringently self-impose quality, potency, and research standards for their products, while others do not. These companies often make their products available only through health care providers, as a means to assure that their products are used effectively. Here are some pointers when using probiotics:

- Use high potency. Make sure the product you choose offers at least 8 billion CFUs (colony forming units) per serving. Some store-bought probiotics are too low potency to be effective.
- Chewable probiotic tablets are often too low potency for therapeutic benefit. If your child likes them, make sure they deliver more viable probiotic than filler ingredients, and that fillers do not contain gluten or other items you may be avoiding.
- Start low, go slow. Infants can start with 4 or 5 billion CFUs per day and increase gradually to whatever level helps them have better stools and sleep, and less colic, diaper rash, and spit-up.
- Children can start at 8 billion CFUs and gradually increase to a level that improves their bowel habits. Some children need 20–40 billion CFUs daily during therapeutic dosing.
- Babies need Bifido strains (like *Bifido infantis*, *Bifido bifidum*, *Bifido breve*) and *Lactobacillus acidophilus*, which are among the first organisms that typically colonize the human gut.
- After age two or three, different strains of Lactobacillus (thermophilus, casei, rhamnosus, and others) may become more important while Bifido strains become less dominant.
- Infants or children with lactic acid excess may need to avoid high doses of probiotics that produce lactic acid, like *Lactobacillus acidophilus*, *L. buchnori*, *L. fementi*, *L. plantarum*, or *L. salivarius*. They can use other strains like Bifido species or *L. rhamnosus*. High lactic acid levels show up on urine organic acid panels or with blood tests.

- *Saccharomcyes boulardii* is a strain of yeast that does not colonize the human gut, but it can be used to aggressively crowd out yeast that is resident there. *S. boulardii* has been clinically reviewed for its effectiveness against intestinal candidiasis and in reducing diarrhea in children. Try this probiotic if your child has fungal overgrowth but medication is not an option.
- Use probiotics following any antibiotic treatment for your child. If your child must use ongoing antibiotics daily, try a product that combines *S. boulardii* with some beneficial strains. Talk to your doctor about minimizing antibiotic therapy if possible.

Bowel Flora Signs and Symptoms

Whether or not your child had a rough start scenario that included lots of antibiotics or feeding tubes, restoring healthy intestinal flora will optimize digestive health, absorption, and immune function, as well as all your efforts with nutrition measures. First, identify if your child needs balancing for bowel flora with the signs and symptoms below. If your child has a normal, brown, formed bowel movement daily with no struggle, and has never had any of these signs or symptoms persist, you can move on to lab work to fully screen for intestinal flora imbalances. They can be present, and treatable, even when these clinical signs are not very active.

If any one of these signs has been persisting long enough to notably irritate your child, then it is likely that yeast or disruptive bacterial bowel flora are part of the problem. Even if your child's bowel movements seem entirely normal, intestinal candidiasis or overgrowth of suboptimal bacterial strains in the gut can produce many irritating symptoms. For example, a young girl came to me with constipation, sudden onset of urine incontinence, and itchy rash on

Clinical Signs for Imbalanced Bowel Flora: Bowel Habits

- Frequent diarrhea, loose wet stool, gold stool, green stool
- Irritable stools that alternate between hard/dry mixed with mushy wet stool
- Constipation (less than one stool per day) that has persisted long enough to need laxatives
- More than three stools per day for more than a month
- Explosive stools, large stools (enough to clog the toilet), exceedingly foul-smelling stools
- Poorly digested food visible in stool on a regular basis
- Any history of these signs lasting more than four months
- Onset of urine or stool incontinence in previously potty trained children

Clinical Signs for Imbalanced Bowel Flora: Behavior

- Mood/behavior swings, tantrums, or extreme irritability, worst when child is hungry
- Sensory irritability, especially for noise
- Silly, suddenly happy, or hyperactive after eating a starchy meal
- Appetite rigid for starchy foods, narrow food choices

Clinical Signs for Imbalanced Bowel Flora: Physical Features and History

- Ringworm rash (coin-size red circles with pale centers)
- Intermittent diffuse rashes of unknown origin
- Acne
- History of oral thrush, needing gentian violet, antifungal treatment for toe or fingernails
- Persisting diaper rash, especially raw or itchy rash
- Bloated belly

her thighs and bottom. The girl needed to urinate more frequently and lost her ability to anticipate needing to use the bathroom—and began having embarrassing accidents at school. After making sure her pediatrician ruled out juvenile diabetes (for which new frequent urination is a classic sign), we did a urine screen for metabolites of yeast, which I suspected because of the nature of the rash and her history of antibiotic use. The test was positive. In this case, the pediatrician decided not to treat the yeast, which could have been triggering all her symptoms, but to give the girl more Miralax—a Band-Aid approach for one symptom only.

In cases like this where a prescription antifungal may have done the trick quick, but you don't get one, you can safely add naturopathic supports to eradicate yeast and improve bowel flora. While there are safe and effective antifungal medications for infants and children, pediatricians will often defer them if they do not believe that yeast is problematic, or when they have limited experience with it. They also must weigh the need for the medication against organism resistance, a problem that has evolved with antibiotics. In other words, they need to save the big guns for the worst situations, so fungal organisms (yeasts) do not acquire resistance to our arsenal of medications. Here are some options to improve bowel flora, based on your cost limitations and provider's advice:

1. Refine the findings for signs and symptoms with lab studies. This is usually a stool culture for strains of yeast and bacteria, or a urine screen that looks for signature chemicals from disruptive yeasts and bowel bacteria. Then work with your provider to pick a targeted treatment based on the new information.
2. Begin high-potency probiotic supplement. As noted earlier, start low and go slow. If your child is already monitored and on a special diet, or has seizures, let your provider know you'd like to try probiotics.

3. Begin naturopathic antifungal herbs and supplements. Check with a naturopath or your doctor if medications are already in the picture to be sure of no cross-sensitivities or reactions.

4. If symptoms are severe enough, or haven't resolved with naturopathic supports like probiotics and herbal antifungals, see if your provider will begin antifungal medication. Dosing has to be high enough and for long enough duration to be effective. Be sure to finish the medication, just as you are advised to do with an antibiotic, even if your child quickly improves. This will reduce likelihood of organism resistance to the drug.

Lab Tests That Identify Bowel Flora Problems

What they are: Providers use stool culture, urine microbial organic acids, and breath tests to identify bowel flora problems.

When to use them: Treatments can almost always begin based on signs and symptoms alone. Use lab studies when you need to identify an effective therapeutic agent, or when you need to confirm the presence of a specific strain of yeast or bacteria.

Where to get them: Doctor's Data and Great Plains Laboratory do the necessary sensitivity and specificity testing on stool samples to identify therapeutic agents for Candida overgrowth. They also will culture for the presence of helpful bacteria in a stool sample, which can tell you if a supplemental probiotic is taking residence as it should in your child's bowel. Your pediatrician's testing tools can confirm the presence of some bowel pathogens such as Clostridia (stool culture) or *Helicobacter pylori* (breath test).

STOOL CULTURE

A stool culture uses a sample of your child's stool, usually collected at home and placed in a special container for delivery to the lab. The lab puts small smears of the stool sample in "media" (usually a type of gelatin with vitamins in it) that support healthful or harmful bacteria. Whatever grows well is then known to be present in your child's bowel. Knowing which strains of yeast or detrimental bacteria are growing helps the provider choose a medication or naturopathic treatment. Some labs also do "sensitivity" testing, in which the strain of bad flora that grew is then killed using several different agents. Some agents do the job, some don't, and this gives still more information for the provider to work with. It lets the provider target the treatment with an agent that is known to be effective for your child's culture.

For stool cultures, biomedical providers typically use specialty labs (Doctors Data or Great Plains Lab) that do this type of sensitivity testing. These labs will also routinely look for beneficial flora in the sample, not just the bad stuff. This indicates whether a child needs probiotics, what kind of dose, what strains, or whether the probiotics you are using are doing any good. It also indicates whether your child's bowel simply can't tolerate beneficial flora, a scenario I have encountered frequently in children with autism. If supplemental probiotics have been relentlessly unsuccessful for a child, it is time to move on to other strategies. You will know if your probiotic is unsuccessful if you've dosed it at at least 10 billion CFUs daily for months or years, and the strain won't culture on a stool test. Or, if your child still shows positive signs for bowel flora problems, it probably isn't working. Have your clinician rule out other more pathogenic bacteria, viruses, or parasites, or whether ongoing use of a reflux medication is interfering with the pH of the bowel and thus making it hard for healthy bacteria to grow.

Conventional stool culture tests used by much of mainstream medicine (your pediatrician or hospital) often have less sensitivity and specificity. They may report a result for Candida (yeast) as "normal" and give no other information. Candida is indeed a normal resident of the human gut, so its presence on a stool panel is in itself no big deal. But since children with autism have been noted to have Candida overgrowth more often than expected, and since autism features can improve with treatment of this, it makes sense to use the labs that give more information on how to treat it. Knowing what strain of yeast is present (there are dozens), to what extent, and what agent will kill it is valuable information for the treatment plan.

NUANCES IN INTERPRETATION OF STOOL CULTURES. I have observed variation in individual sensitivity to strains of yeast. For example, stool panels that culture *Sacccharomyces cerevisiae* within acceptable limits (noted as 1+ or 2+ on the lab result) seem to coincide with terrible irritability in the child and in stool pattern. It may be that the culture plate was not ideal to grow that strain in numbers that reflect its presence in the child's gut—in any case, my opinion is that this be treated as though it is an overgrowth situation. Also, if a child has active clinical signs for intestinal candidiasis, a urine panel that sees Candida signature chemicals to excess, and a stool culture that says Candida is barely visible, I will assume the culture plate medium was not precisely to the yeast's liking—that is, yeast is there to excess but it simply did not grow well on that particular culture medium. Again, ideally, antifungal treatment will ensue. It is a generally benign measure unless children are using medications that cannot be mixed with drugs like Diflucan or Sporanox (Nystatin is usually a safe choice in that case), and nearly always triggers positive changes in appetite, stools, bloating, and reflux. It also appears to mitigate sound sensitivity, sensory irritability, and oral tactile defensiveness, and in some cases improves expressive language.

HOW TO COLLECT A STOOL SAMPLE AT HOME. I get asked this a lot. Most kids don't mind peeing in a cup, but for the other business, I haven't yet met one who wants to offer up a sample in this way! If your child is out of diapers and uses the toilet instead of a potty, here's a trick to keep him oblivious to what you are doing—useful for children with anxiety or who have already been through a lot with regard to potty training. Your child does not need to know that you are collecting a stool sample, if this works best for him. Or inform him if that works, knowing that he only needs information that he asks for, and probably less. Drain most of the water out of your toilet bowl by turning off the valve behind the toilet. Then secure a low-slung, plastic wrap hammock across the back half of the bowl, and close the seat. This lets urine run into the bowl in the front, and catches stool on the "hammock" toward the back. Ideally, urine should not mix with stool for best results on a stool sample. Lift the sample-laden hammock out of the toilet and process it per your lab kit instructions.

Urine Screens for Imbalanced Bowel Flora

This is a test that looks for organic acids rarely produced in human metabolism but known to be produced by certain disruptive bacteria, such as Clostridia, or yeast. It looks for their signature chemicals—chemicals only made by those substances. The test is called a Microbial OAT (organic acid test) and usually includes a panel of several organic acids. High levels imply that something other than your child is producing these acids; the acids are circulated systemically, including in the brain; and the acids are very likely caused by bowel flora your child would be better off without. This test is like finding the smoking gun and not the culprit itself. It does not culture the microbial strain itself and thus can't predict which agents will kill it. But it can be an easy way to screen whether or not gut dysbiosis (imbalanced flora) is a problem. It is especially helpful when there are minimal clinical signs for bowel problems, but ample behavior signs. Many parents won't go through with stool sample collection if bowel movements or GI symptoms are not terribly problematic for a child, but they are willing to do an easy urine screen.

BREATH TEST FOR BOWEL FLORA

One particularly disruptive bacteria, *Helicobacter pylori*, can be detected by a simple breath test. This bacteria can infect the stomach or upper small intestine, and can cause ulcers, gastritis, or increase risk for cancer. A gastroenterologist can determine if this is a needed test, or whether further screenings for this kind of infection are appropriate. Children with autism spectrum disorders, so far, do not appear to have *H. pylori* infection more often than typical peers, but if this is present, treating it will make your child healthier and more comfortable.

Optimizing Bowel Flora

Once you know bowel flora status for your child, treatment should ensue posthaste. Bear in mind that if your pediatrician thought this was a good idea, he would have prescribed treatment long ago. Current pediatric practice generally permits antifungal treatment when a child has visible signs of thrush or candidiasis, that is, when there is a white velvety coating on the tongue, lips, anus, or genitals. In other words, unless yeast is literally coming out of your child at both ends, treatment may not be offered. One child with autism in my caseload had candidiasis so entrenched for so many years that yeast was visibly coming out of his ears. This caused deafness to a degree that he now uses hearing aids.

Children showing signs of trouble per the list above can be treated successfully well before the problem gets this bad. I have watched many a nutrition intervention skewered by foot-dragging on this piece. Since disruptive flora can gobble up B vitamins, other vitamins or minerals, and even some amino acids, some children react quite adversely when supplements are begun before this piece is adequately treated. How does this look? Your child may show extreme irritability, insomnia, reactivity, violent behavior, or hyperactivity when given the supplements he may need to function and feel better. All these goodies fertilize the bowel flora, which then excrete enough toxins to overwhelm the liver's capacity to manage them, and boom— they are in brain tissue, affecting behavior, mood, and so on. Children who show persisting hypersensitivity to supplements or medications may still be struggling with really disruptive bowel flora. Untreated bowel imbalances can also keep progress on a special diet slow and frustrating. A sure sign of this is when there is little change in appetite rigidity after months using gluten-free, casein-free foods. Here are the tools for the job:

Probiotics

As discussed earlier, young infants can use probiotics and there are preparations just for them. Bifido bacteria with a little Lactobacillus is a good blend for this age (up to one year old), as it is one of the first bacteria that normally populates the newborn gut. You can dust a bottle or breast nipple with probiotic powder to start, and watch for tolerance. Infants older than six months can use probiotic powder, to a quarter teaspoon, in soft foods. This has a mildly sweet taste not too different from cotton candy, even though it is unsweetened. Toddlers can shift to blends that emphasize Lactobacillus and other strains. Some children do well with high-potency single-strain preparations such as Culturelle; others never do, and need blends of six or eight beneficial strains instead. Stool cultures can help inform at the start, but observing your child's demeanor, feeding, and stool patterns is a good barometer, too. A formed, easy to eliminate, uniform brown stool daily is a sign that things are improving.

Older children who have gut dysbiosis need higher potencies of probiotic, starting in the range of 8–10 billion "colony forming units" (CFUs) per dose, perhaps twice a day. Some children do better on much more, at 20–40 billion CFUs per day. Start at the lowest dose, observe, and increase to a therapeutic dose gradually. Check labels for dosage. Labels that give doses in grams or milligrams, and not in colony forming units, are difficult to discern for effectiveness since there is no way to tell how many active units of beneficial flora are present. There may be fillers in these that are not beneficial. Chewable probiotic tablets and eating yogurt daily are healthy habits for typical situations, but they can't deliver the effective doses of probiotic needed to kill off or crowd out unwanted microbes. Children with casein intolerance cannot use yogurt made with dairy products, so appropriate supplementation becomes more important.

ANTIFUNGALS

There are prescription medications for fungal infections and intestinal candidiasis, as well as many naturopathic agents. Prescriptions can include Nystatin, Diflucan, Sporanox, Nizoral, or their generic counterparts. As with antibiotics, there is always a concern that repeat use of these drugs may help a yeast strain acquire resistance to it. Hence it is important to finish a prescription completely, even if symptoms you are treating have resolved. Rotation with antifungal herbs or supplements can help keep yeast from returning. There are several: calendula, oregano oil, goldenseal, uva ursi (use for only 4 to 7 days at a time), garlic, tea tree, black walnut, pau d'arco, monolaurin, cranberry extract, grapefruit seed extract, olive leaf extract, caprylic acid, and more. These are available in various forms, from capsules and powders to liquid tinctures, individually or as blends. Which ones you might use may depend on your child's stool culture sensitivity panel, tolerance, or ease of use. Herb tinctures in glycerite are great for children because they are easy to use: Mix the dose in an ounce or so of water in a paper cup. Some are bitter and some are pleasant. Companies such as Herbs for Kids, WishGarden, and HerbPharm make preparations that can treat candidiasis. Always use new items like this at a time when you can observe your child for a few hours, to watch for any complications—not right before bed, and not right before school, but on a quiet morning at home when you can observe, or when your child is with a trusted care provider who will report any changes to you.

Another item that has shown clinical effectiveness in reducing intestinal candidiasis and correcting chronic diarrhea in children is a strain of nonpathogenic yeast called *Saccharomyces boulardii*, or *S. boulardii* for short. This yeast does not like to take up residence in the human gut, but will work to reduce levels of pathogenic flora, for as long as it is supplemented. Data on ideal duration of use is scant, but my observation is that this works for about a 30-day period. After that, it's probably time to put a new item in the antifungal rotation. Some supplements contain *Saccharomyces cerevisiae*, which is a strain of yeast that can reside in the human gut. I have observed this strain to be quite disruptive in small children even when cultured within a normal range on a stool sample. For children with gut dysbiosis, it is probably prudent to avoid *S. cerevisiae* in supplements.

A FINAL NOTE. Individuals vary greatly with respect to how Candida or other strains of yeast seem to affect them. This may relate to how toxins from these microbes are managed in children with autism or learning and psychiatric diagnoses (back to methylation, transsulfuration, or paths in liver tissue that detoxify stuff). In any case, when a child has visible clinical signs for yeast and the lab panels say all is well, I treat the signs and symptoms, not the lab panel. The old adage "look at the kid" applies here. Sometimes yeast does not culture well on the stool panel but it shows up as a smoking gun on the urine panel. Treat it. Sometimes both panels show levels of yeast within an acceptable reference range, but the child is struggling with active signs and symptoms. Treat it. In these cases, you will only know if it helps once you try it.

How Can You Tell
If Bowel Flora Is Repaired?

Back to signs and symptoms. If your child is not showing any of the issues in that bullet list for bowel flora signs and symptoms, you are probably there. You could repeat lab testing at this point if you like, but it is usually not necessary. If you've gotten these signs and symptoms as well controlled as possible with antifungal treatments and probiotics, but there are still problems, it's time for Step 3 in your child's nutrition care process: Replace foods that are not tolerated with equal or better nutritional value. If you've already begun this by withdrawing a couple of suspect foods, but symptoms for intolerance are still active, then you should proceed with lab tests that can clarify what is triggering the inflammation. If you are enjoying a stretch of calm in this regard—and your child is eating, sleeping, eliminating, playing, learning, and behaving better—put your feet up, celebrate this success, and dive in with new foods and suggestions in Chapter 6.

Lab Tests for Food Allergy, Sensitivity, and Intolerance

There are several reasons to look into food allergy, sensitivity, and intolerance after you check into bowel flora. At the top of the list is the fact that children with autism have already been noted for having food allergy, sensitivity, and intolerance more often than typical peers, in a number of research trials (these are referenced in my learning module, "Medical Nutrition Therapy for Pediatric Autism"; see "Resources and Further Reading"). I find that children with sensory integration disorder reliably do, too, based on those I've encountered and tested myself. As noted earlier, children with autism also are noted to have intestinal candidiasis too often. How does this relate to food allergy? First, if there are problems like ongoing intestinal candidiasis, then your child is likely to have a food allergy, sensitivity, and/or intolerance (each is distinct from the other, and is explained in the coming pages) because intestinal candidiasis can create leaky gut syndrome (intestinal permeability). Yeast overgrowth in the gut takes to tissue there a little like ivy can take to the mortar in a chimney—it roots itself and actually penetrates a bit. This means the intestine becomes more porous and less selective about molecular fragments and toxins that are allowed to pass into the body. So you need healthy bowel flora to prevent or repair a "leaky" gut.

Food allergy, sensitivity, and intolerance can trigger inflammation in gut tissue itself by physically damaging the delicate structures in there, by flooding spaces made for absorbing tiny food molecules with white blood cells (this is called "esoinphilia in crypts" on an endoscopy report); or systemically, by triggering the immune system to make antibodies to things it doesn't really need to worry about (such as food proteins). Meanwhile, an inflamed gut can make an unwelcome environment for beneficial flora—one of the tools you need to fix the problem. This means you will need to withdraw inflammatory foods and use safe, nutritious, non-inflammatory alternatives. New foods that you introduce will not be well tolerated in a leaky gut, because they will simply stream into circulation in forms that trigger new immune responses, causing more inflammation for your child. This is why children who are dairy-protein intolerant don't often succeed with a soy milk replacement—if the gut is "leaky," the soy protein is soon able to trigger the same problems for inflammation as the dairy protein did. It's best to begin balancing bowel flora ahead of rotating in new food, and use an amino acid–based formula as a milk substitute at first if possible—more on that in Chapter 5.

As soon as bowel flora is optimized, the leaky gut can begin to recover, and new foods can be rotated in. It's not reasonable or safe to withdraw every food that shows an inflammatory response for your child, but the biggest food triggers for inflammation must be withdrawn completely. Lab tests can help clarify this, but again are not an absolute to begin a diet trial. Signs and symptoms can often yield enough information to begin. When you feel you need more, lab tests can fill in the blanks. These tests can help you with Step 3, replacing foods in your child's diet. You need to know which foods are best tolerated and which ones will worsen inflammation or irritability.

What the tests are: Providers typically use RAST or ELISA tests to identify immune responses to foods. They use urine polypeptide analysis to identify digestive (not immune) intolerance to wheat and dairy proteins.

When to use them: When it is too hard to identify trigger foods with elimination diets; when you need proof of circulating antibodies/inflammation triggered by an offending food; when you need proof of immune reactions to wheat and dairy proteins.

Where to get them: While conventional pediatric allergists administer RAST tests for classic food allergy (IgE), many do not acknowledge or use ELISA tests, which measure a different immune response (technically, a food "sensitivity") that is mediated more slowly (IgG). ELISA testing is done by most biomedical providers and is available from Great Plains Lab, Doctor's Data, York Labs, ImmunoLabs, or Metamatrix Labs. A pediatric gastroenterologist may also be able to order IgG sensitivities tests for some foods, and celiac panels sometimes include IgG testing for gluten sensitivity. Specialty labs listed here can test dozens of food sensitivities with one 2-millimeter tube of blood or even a tiny "capillary" tube—a vast improvement over drawing the four tubes that were once required.

Although parents usually cringe the most at the idea of having to withdraw and replace a food in a child's diet, it is probably the easiest part. Identifying problem foods is not that difficult, once the lab options are well understood. There are also many fantastic substitutes now for wheat and dairy foods, alternatives that did not exist when I first took this on in 1997. There are essentially three paths to tread in order to identify foods that are problematic for a child with autism spectrum concerns, ADHD, or learning and psychiatric diagnoses: food allergy, food sensitivity, and food intolerance. They are distinct from each other, according to the American Academy of Allergy and Immunology Committee on Adverse Reactions to Foods (detailed explanations follow their definitions below):

- Food allergy is anaphylaxis—that is, an allergic reaction that occurs immediately and systemically. It involves immunoglobulin E (IgE) and swift release of other immune chemicals such as histamine. Signs of anaphylaxis can include acute and sudden onset of hives, wheezing, vomiting, abdominal pain or cramps, or diarrhea, following ingestion of the trigger food.
- Food sensitivity is an immune reaction to a food, usually delayed, that may not involve IgE but may involve immunoglobulin G (IgG).
- Food intolerance is an abnormal physiologic response to a food, including idiosyncratic, metabolic, pharmacologic, or toxic reactions.

FOOD ALLERGIES

These are anaphylactic reactions to foods, the kind that require an EpiPen to treat immediately. Life-threatening food allergies in children have risen dramatically since the mid-1980s. It's usually easy to see when this is brewing for a child. There will be obvious and fast signs of trouble: hives, vomiting, swelling. This kind of reaction to a food can be identified with a skin prick test or a blood test that can be done by a conventional pediatric allergist. If it is highly positive, your child should eliminate the offending food. Children with asthma and chronic infections are especially likely to feel much better when they avoid IgE trigger foods. In my experience, doing this permits children with asthma to use less medication, including inhalers, steroids, antihistamines, or drugs such as Zyrtec, and slows or stops the merry-go-round of repeat ear or upper respiratory infections. If your child has asthma, reducing inflammatory load from foods is a relatively easy thing to do, and it can make for fewer episodes of asthma, flu, colds, and emergency room visits.·

FOOD SENSITIVITIES

IgE testing can be entirely negative while other immune reactions to foods can be active and positive. If your child has had food allergy testing and you were told it was negative, but there are still chronic inflammatory symptoms (asthma, wheezing, colds, cough, eczema, irritable stools), you need to do further testing for food *sensitivities*. IgE testing only checks for classic food allergy, not sensitivities. This is a slower immune response, usually mediated by a different molecule made by the body, called immunoglobulin G (IgG). This is by far the more common problem in my practice, for two reasons: First, these reactions often go undetected; signs and symptoms are more gradual and insidious, making them harder to relate to food. And second, these reactions often go undetected because the proper way to test for them has been a subject of debate. While a pediatrician will often make a referral for classic allergy testing, it is much less common for "sensitivity" testing to be permitted. Some allergists are unsure how to do it; others don't acknowledge that food sensitivities matter or that the testing for them is useful. A test called Enzyme Linked Immunosorbent Assay (ELISA) is popular in the biomedical treatment community for this. It requires blood draw; most labs that do this test have refined it to the point where one 2-milliliter tube of blood can be used to check IgG reactions to some 90 foods. There are saliva and finger stick tests for this also, giving parents several options for testing.

Clinical trials have shown ELISA to be as effective as a rotation or elimination diet in predicting which foods are problematic. These diets withdraw a suspected offending food, then reintroduce it a few weeks later; you wait to see how you feel on and off the food. For years this was proffered as the best tool for children to use for sorting out trigger foods. For the population of kids discussed in this book, rotation and elimination diets are not a very good option. They take too long, especially for children struggling with growth deficits who need to restore food intakes as quickly as possible, and they are hard for parents to comply with when more than two foods are in question, which is usually true for the kids I encounter. Waiting months to identify a therapeutic diet strategy is not a reasonable option, and neither is open-ended dependence on medications that treat symptoms of food intolerance (irritable stools, constipation, reflux, anxiety, frequent colds and coughs, intermittent eczema, or asthma/wheezing).

BABIES AND FOOD SENSITIVITIES

IgG sensitivities can begin in infancy and have been shown to impair growth and feeding in infants (see "Resources and Further Reading" for the learning module if you'd like academic reading and referencing on this piece). Babies who struggle with colic, vomiting, spitting up, eczema, crying, mucousy stools, slower than expected growth velocity, and poor sleep should be tested to rule out an immune sensitivity to milk protein (casein IgG). Since the immune system at this age is so immature, ELISA testing is not appropriate for babies, as the test may show several false positives. For the same reason, careful interpretation of ELISA tests is important when they are used for children under age two. These tests have been used in research settings on infants and children but are not common or even well understood in everyday pediatrics. This age group is one in which an elimination diet can do some diagnostic good, since the only major protein infants and even young toddlers consume is often casein, whether it comes from cow's milk, goat milk, or human milk. A food diary will tell you if this is true in your child's case. If there are several protein sources in the food diary (milk, eggs, meats, chicken, beans, soy), then an elimination diet is cumbersome, slow, and confusing as a diagnostic tool. But if the food diary simply repeats casein in every color of the rainbow (yogurt, cheese, milk, cottage cheese, cheese sticks, cheese crackers, Peptamen Junior, or milk-based infant formulas) with little or no mention of other protein foods ever being eaten, then you can reliably try an elimination diet instead of lab work.

Casein from different mammals is differentiated by subtle molecular configurations, which is why some babies do fine with Mom's breast milk but cannot manage cow's milk. If a newborn has needed antibiotics, or did not tolerate early rounds of shots, the gut may become leaky enough for even Mom's milk to be intolerable. This means that fragments of poorly digested casein molecules are squeaking through the gut and getting into circulation, where they trigger the immune system to react. When this is left untreated, it can escalate into more inflammation from more foods as they are introduced. It's easy to treat early on by giving babies formulas that they can digest better, and by using gentle probiotics.

Some babies who have been given antibiotics may also need antifungal medication to correct things. Semi-elemental formulas (aka "hydrolysates") such as Nutramigen and Alimentum are much better choices in this situation than soy-based formulas, since soy protein can be as difficult for babies to digest as casein. Soy formula is also tougher on the baby's gut because of its higher iron content, which is raised to overcome how soy interferes with iron absorption. If the semi-elemental formulas don't provide fast resolution of symptoms, the next step is to try an elemental formula, also called amino acid–based formula (AABF), such as Neocate. This will usually do the trick, and it permits the intestine to recover by completely eliminating inflammation from intact dietary proteins. AABF has been shown to reverse intestinal permeability in infants and young children with leaky gut syndrome.

A final option is to use goat milk infant formula, since this may be tolerated by babies who can't handle breast milk, hydrolysates, or AABF. See Chapter 6 for a safe goat milk formula for infants, and let your pediatrician know if you want to try it. What you cannot do is use milks from rice, almond, oat, hemp, or nuts for infant formula, nor can you use regular cow's milk, soy milk, yogurt, or smoothie blends. For many reasons, *these are unsafe and inappropriate substitutes for formula or breast milk for infants under a year old.* Once a baby is past four months, yogurt may be a fine addition to the diet along with the usual introduction of solids, as long as cow casein is not a problem for the baby. It often is, which is why my preference is goat yogurt, as goat casein is gentler for an infant's digestion. Check Specific Carbohydrate Diet recipes and recommendations on the Web for a goat yogurt that might be especially easy for babies to digest. With the right feedings, your baby should keep growing, eliminating, exploring, and feeding as expected, and should sleep better, too. Babies will show trouble especially fast by slowing down gains for weight or length—you can always have your pediatrician check this for you.

Since children eat a variety of protein sources by age two and beyond, rotation or elimination diets become cumbersome at that point for sorting out what foods might be triggering symptoms. Some data on children show that they, too, like infants, can experience growth impairment if IgG reactions to foods are chronically active. My observation is that these children often have weak, picky appetites and mixed irritable stools. IgG reactions can inflame intestinal tissue. Though they don't cause a release of histamine as IgE reactions do, they can activate other immune chemicals. IgG reactions take anywhere from an hour or two to a couple of days to trigger effects, which can include reflux, diarrhea, mixed irritable stools, bloating, pain, cramping, fatigue, runny nose, eczema, migraines or headaches, or mood/sensory irritability. A common sign of IgG inflammation from foods is pallor with allergic shiners under the eyes, which may occur due to poor absorption of nutrients such as iron, secondary to inflammation in the intestine. IgG-mediated food sensitivities are also called "delayed allergies." Though they are technically not a classic allergy, their effects can last weeks beyond eating a trigger food. This is why offending foods must be withdrawn for a long time to give a clear indication of functional benefits for a child, and to permit gut tissue recovery.

Should I Cut Gluten from My Child's Diet?

Most parents have now heard of gluten avoidance as a therapeutic measure for autism, diabetes, sensory integration disorder, and other special needs. This is a complex issue, as gluten may cause any one— or all three—of the problems mentioned at the start of this section: allergy, sensitivity, or intolerance. How each may affect your child and how you test for each of these is different, though the treatment would be the same: eliminating gluten.

"Allergy" to gluten is checked with a RAST test, and your pediatrician or pediatric allergist can do this for you. Usually, this involves a blood test or a skin-prick test. This checks IgE level to wheat—and gluten is the protein in wheat. Many children enter my practice with this testing already done. With few exceptions, IgE to wheat is negative and the parent is told gluten is no problem. Certainly, if you find your child has a positive IgE to wheat, it should without question be eliminated, just as you would avoid cat dander or dust mites with a positive IgE to those allergens. Inexplicably, I have encountered children who were not told to avoid wheat even when IgE was highly positive. Obviously, you will not want your child ingesting a known, highly inflammatory food. It can exacerbate inflammatory conditions like asthma or cystic fibrosis and can disrupt behavior, sleep, bowel habits, growth, learning, and mood.

"Sensitivity" to gluten is checked with ELISA IgG panels that include gluten-containing foods like wheat, barley, rye, and oats. These panels sometimes include gliadin also, which is a component of the gluten molecule. A gliadin IgG test is highly specific for gluten sensitivity. Some mainstream pediatric providers or gastroenterologists will order it (usually as part of a celiac screen blood test) or it is available from labs mentioned earlier, such as ImmunoLabs or Great Plains Lab. If it is positive, then your child is likely experiencing systemic, chronic inflammation from gluten, and may experience relief from several symptoms if gluten is avoided.

IgG antibodies to gliadin have been shown to cross-react with brain tissue. This means that when a gluten-sensitive child eats gluten, the IgG antibodies that react to it may mistake brain tissue for gliadin proteins, and attack the brain tissue. Some researchers postulate that this is one reason why individuals with celiac disease often have neurological and psychiatric complications, and why children with autism tend to improve when they avoid gluten. A test for anti-gliadin IgG antibody (available separately, or included in some ELISA panels) can tell you if this is active in your child.

"Intolerance" to gluten means that there is not necessarily any immune response to it, but it is not tolerated because of other problems. In autism, gluten intolerance may fall under what researchers call the Opiate Theory, explained in more detail later in this chapter. In this scenario, gluten is not digested enough by enzymes in the GI tract, and it is absorbed in the wrong form—that is, as an oversize peptide molecule that can lock on to endorphin receptors in the brain, where it impairs speech, cognition, behavior, sleep, and mood. Casein may create the same insult—thus the progress seen with gluten- and casein-avoidance diets.

CLEARING THE CONFUSION:
WHAT CELIAC DISEASE AND GLUTEN INTOLERANCE HAVE TO DO WITH AUTISM

Celiac disease is a condition in which gluten—the protein in grains such as wheat, rye, barley, or oats—triggers a chronic immune response. In celiac disease, chronic inflammation triggered by gluten eventually destroys the intestinal lining so much that food cannot be absorbed. Usually, but not always, children with true celiac will show at least one of these obvious clinical signs: growth regression or growth failure, stomach pain, headaches, frequent illness, anemia, poor concentration or mood problems, and chronic diarrhea/irritable stools. Many children grow up undiagnosed with celiac disease and do not find relief until adulthood, when a diagnosis is finally made. Persons with celiac disease are treated with a gluten-free diet, and most of the time, this reverses the disease process. Eating gluten will further the disease process, and can increase risk for certain cancers. Therefore, it is best treated as early as possible.

Currently in the United States, many gastroenterologists regard celiac disease as the only rationale for a gluten-free diet in a child. Some do not believe that gluten sensitivity matters or exists, outside of true celiac disease. Tests that screen for celiac disease look for autoantibodies to gut tissue that develop only in celiac disease. These are tissue trans-glutaminase antibody, reticulin antibody, and endomysial antibody. To find out if your child is gluten sensitive, you need an IgG antigliadin antibody test, not a celiac screening test. A negative celiac test does not mean that your child tolerates gluten. It simply means your child does not have celiac disease.

If you have received a positive celiac test for your child, further testing can confirm the diagnosis, and a gastroenterologist can guide you on this. Genetic testing, skin biopsy, or gut biopsy are ways that a diagnosis of celiac disease can be confirmed. In an effort to follow up on initial findings about damaged gut tissue in children with autism, some researchers have explored whether this damage is in fact celiac disease. The answer appears to be no, and data from my own caseload matches what others are finding so far: that children with autism have positive antigliadin antibodies more often than typical peers, but they do not have celiac disease. In the general population, only about 10 percent of people will have a positive gliadin antibody. So far, children with autism appear to have this closer to 70 to 80 percent of the time. In other words, children with autism are usually gluten-sensitive and experience inflammation from gluten, but they do not have celiac disease. This means they may well improve by eliminating gluten from their diets, even when they don't have celiac disease. Overwhelmingly, my own experience with hundreds of children in this boat is that they do improve with gluten-free diets.

Even with distinct tests for celiac disease and gluten sensitivity, confusion still abounds. A positive antigliadin antibody finding is often construed as a "false positive" when a child does not also have celiac disease, and a parent will be told that all the results are normal. This is because gastroenterologists in the United States are currently trained to regard gluten sensitivity as probably not relevant, outside of true celiac disease. If you've done this panel, ask to see the actual lab results yourself. If the panel did not include the gliadin IgG antibody, you need another blood test to look at that. If it did, and if the result was above the reference range or high in the normal range, your child may be a candidate for a gluten-free diet. The reason is that in my experience, children vary with the degree to which antigliadin antibody irritates them or interferes with growth and functioning. One child age two whom I met showed an antigliadin IgG result of 19, with above 20 being considered out of range. This toddler met nutritional failure criteria because he had not grown in a year and was about to begin growth hormone injections. The family was told that gluten was not a factor, based on this lab finding. Given other active signs and symptoms for this child, including the growth delay, autism diagnosis, neurological signs such as ataxia and nystagmus, and messy wet stools, I encouraged a gluten-free trial first. It was so successful that the child remained gluten-free for several years, grew well, and eventually lost the autism diagnosis—a diagnosis that was quite appropriate at the time of my initial consult with this child. No growth hormone was needed.

By contrast, I have also encountered a typically developing, socially engaged child with highly elevated antigliadin antibody and no signs of growth delay, bowel concerns, or frank neurological signs other than some difficulty with focus in school, mood, and athletic pursuits. In this case, the parent wanted to try going gluten-free to see if it would ease learning, athletics, and school stresses. These two cases illustrate once again why *lab data alone does not provide enough information for nutrition care planning.* Every child is different, and individualized care will accommodate these differences for the best outcomes.

MULTIPLE FOOD ALLERGIES OR INTOLERANCE

What if your child is reactive to several foods? The most common trigger foods in children I have tested are without question dairy foods (casein and whey proteins), wheat, and gluten-containing grains (wheat, barley, rye, oat). These frequently display high to very high reactivity on IgG sensitivity panels. Some children show IgE sensitivity to these as well, though this is less frequent in my experience. Invariably, benefits ensue from avoiding these proteins, as long as the diet remains adequate for total protein intake and bowel flora are treated. Benefits do not ensue quickly, if at all, if the child's diet becomes too low for total calories or total protein, if other common trigger proteins are substituted (such as soy) while the gut is still inflamed, or if bowel flora remains problematic.

What about children whose panels come back looking like a Vegas boulevard—completely lit up? This is not unusual for the "one in six" children, and it seems to generally worsen as the developmental, learning, or psychiatric diagnosis becomes more severe. In these cases, four, six, or as many as eight major protein sources are highly reactive, followed by dozens with moderate or low reactivity. The best way to manage this situation is to work in the context of the child's signs and symptoms, and prioritize by choosing up to three, perhaps four, major offender foods to eliminate, and rotate the rest. If the child feels well, is growing well, has no obvious bowel signs, does not have a major developmental or learning handicap, and is not challenged by mood or behavior problems, perhaps pick one food to withdraw and note if any improvement is triggered in a four-to-six-month period. Some children will find it easier to focus and concentrate with this measure. If a child has a major developmental, learning, or behavior diagnosis, and clinical signs are highly active for sensory, mood, and stool irritability, then it makes sense to withdraw more foods to reduce the inflammatory load. Priority is given to foods that are highly IgE reactive. For example, if eggs show high reactivity mediated by both IgE and IgG, then eggs should go on the strict elimination list, at least for the first four months. Two other proteins may then be chosen—most likely, gluten and casein.

In my opinion, it is not feasible or advisable to withdraw several major proteins from a child's diet at once. The diet becomes too restrictive and children tend to struggle to eat enough. I have met many families trying to avoid every food indicated on an ELISA panel, and typically, it is an uphill battle that is not yielding enough benefit to continue. A great option in this situation is to use AABF formulated for children. This is discussed in detail in Chapter 5.

Food Intolerance

What the lab test is: Urine Polypeptide Analysis or Gluten Casein Peptide Test (urine).

When to use it: Use this to confirm excess formation of dietary opiates for a child with autism, aphasia, or language delays.

Where to get it: AAL Reference Labs, Great Plains Lab.

Other than reactions to foods mediated by the immune system, intolerance is another category of reactions in itself. Most people are familiar with lactose intolerance, for example. Lactose is the sugar (carbohydrate) in milk. If you lack the enzyme to break it down, as most adults across the world do, you will experience bloating, gas, and diarrhea. This is not an immune response, and it has nothing to do with casein (the protein) in milk, which is why children on casein-free diets cannot use lactose-free milk. Lactose-free milk still has protein in it, and lactase enzyme drops or pills won't make a dent in how the protein is absorbed.

It's not unusual for a milk protein sensitivity to be mistaken for lactose intolerance in children, because the initial symptoms are similar. However, allergy or sensitivity to milk protein will usually trigger symptoms that last longer, up to weeks, where as lactose intolerance resolves in a day or two after withdrawing dairy food. Allergic shiners under the eyes, rashes, and mood irritability or anxiety are features of an IgG-mediated immune response that would not be typical of simple lactose intolerance.

This is where the Opiate Theory comes into the discussion, which is a big piece of the autism puzzle. This is an example of a food intolerance, not an immune response. It is an inability to normally digest proteins in wheat and dairy foods. Besides active immune responses to wheat and dairy foods, children with autism frequently show an inability to digest these foods. In this scenario, wheat and dairy proteins are partly broken down into molecules called polypeptides, instead of being adequately digested into smaller molecules (peptides and amino acids). These polypeptides normally would not be able to cross the intestinal wall, but children with autism often have intestines that are too permeable or "leaky." This lets these molecules loose into circulation, where they are free to travel to the brain and exert their effects. Low digestive enzyme output conspires with leaky gut to allow a majority of wheat and dairy proteins (gluten and casein) to be absorbed in the wrong form, a form that locks firmly onto endorphin receptors in the brain.

It has been understood for decades that humans don't digest protein completely, and that we usually leave about 10 percent of a protein meal as polypeptide in the gut. These polypeptides are thus more rare in a healthy intestine, and less likely to be absorbed when they are present. In autism, the Opiate Theory suggests that most of the time, protein meals are *mostly* absorbed as polypeptide through a leaky gut.

These molecules resemble opiates, and trigger effects similar to opiate compounds: high pain sensitivity, constipation, cognitive impairments, and blocking of expressive language. Opiate-like compounds from foods are called dietary opiates. They interfere with normal neurotransmitter chemistry by barging in on normal endogenous opiate function (anyone who has heard of endorphins, or who has experienced a positive, contented feeling after exercise or meditation, knows how endogenous endorphins feel). Dietary opiates are also highly addictive, which is why children with autism tend to have extremely rigid, self-restricted diets. They are literally addicted to what they eat, and will vehemently refuse variety.

When these foods are removed, a withdrawal period often ensues in which a child's behavior will dramatically worsen. This may not appear for a week or two, since dietary opiates engaged at endorphin receptors take a long while to leave. Many parents are delighted to find that at the very start of a gluten-free, casein-free diet, their child takes quickly to allowed versions of their old favorites. I somewhat dread the happy phone calls that often ensue at this point from families—things are about to get harder and I hate to rain on the parade. Usually about a week to ten days later, the child will begin refusing most foods offered as he settles on a hunger strike, waiting it out, testing parents' mettle, to see if the opiate-rich versions of his meals will return. This is a daunting time for all, but it can and does pass, and children emerge all the better in most cases. Tricks to survive it and enhance success are discussed in Chapter 6.

It can be daunting to have high hopes for removing wheat and dairy foods, when doing so just seems to cause more trouble. You can avoid this by working with an experienced provider, instead of going it alone. Removing these two proteins can uncover new problems—like peeling layers of an onion—which need treatment in themselves. Many parents stop here after tinkering with gluten-free, casein-free foods, and assert, "The diet didn't work for us." If your child went from constipation to messy loose stools off wheat and dairy, this implies inflammation from foods that was hidden by the constipating effect of dietary opiates, and/or untreated gut dysbiosis. Back to Steps 1 and 2: First, check if your child's growth and food intakes are as expected, and second, make sure you've balanced bowel flora. While it's okay to continue a restricted diet as you revisit these first steps, I place these first in the sequence of special diet tools because skipping these steps will disrupt nutrition measures that follow. They need to come first, and this usually puts the intervention back on track.

How do you know if dietary opiates are active? Urine polypeptide testing is available, but this is regarded as an entirely novel tool and so it is not covered by insurance—expect to pay for it. Polypeptides from gluten and casein, called gluteomorphin (or gliadorphin, gliadomorphin) and casomorphin, are detectable in urine. Generally, it appears that the more profound the autism diagnosis, the more opiate is found in urine. Children with Asperger's syndrome show this less often. That said, a negative finding for opiates does not mean your child can eat gluten and casein, because there may still be immune responses occurring. Urine polypeptide testing does not detect immune responses to food proteins.

A final caveat on urine polypeptide testing: If only one dietary opiate is positive in urine, I recommend that parents withdraw both gluten and casein. This is because wheat and dairy proteins rely on the same set of enzymes in the gut for digestion. One polypeptide being positive while the other is within normal range in urine may simply reflect the child's preference for wheat or dairy protein in his food intake, not an ability to digest one over the other. If the food diary reveals that dairy protein is by far the one the child eats, you may see casomorphin to be positive on the urine panel while gluteomorphin is not. This means that once dairy foods are withdrawn, the child will likely to shift his preference to gluten, since an opiate will likely form with that as well. Children who do this do not show progress to the same degree as children who withdraw both proteins, but many parents will do only what labs tell them. This is a reminder of why it is important to apply findings from the whole assessment picture, and not just lab data, to succeed with special diet interventions. If you have withdrawn only one of these proteins for a child with an autism spectrum diagnosis, including Asperger's syndrome, signs that you should remove both are persisting problems with speech, reciprocal conversation, or understanding social context; persisting constipation or irritable stools; or persisting dietary rigidity and ongoing refusal of new foods.

Parents usually want to know if withdrawing gluten and casein is truly necessary, and they hope that the lab results will give them the definitive answer. As is true with every measure discussed in this book, the final test is how your child does once you fully implement it. Labs can offer some, but not total, predictability. Children who have entirely negative urine polypeptide screens have improved enough with avoidance of gluten and dairy for their families to stick with it. Remember to *piece together the entire picture*—clinical signs and symptoms as well as lab information—to make your choices.

ENZYMES OR AVOIDANCE?

When parents hold out hope to keep wheat or dairy in the picture, I am often asked about enzymes. There are specially formulated supplemental enzymes to break down gluten and casein peptides. When these were first available, they caused quite a stir, and some families found that they got enough benefit just from enzymes to allow their children with autism to eat wheat and dairy foods, rather than using dietary restriction. The drawback is that they must be used at every meal and snack. Because a single molecule of gluten or casein can liberate dozens of opiate-like polypeptides, and based on observation in practice, my opinion is that it works better to use the dietary restriction, especially at first. I advise families to avoid both proteins strictly for a six-month trial period. For goof-ups, have enzymes on hand to minimize release of opiates into circulation, but it is best at first not to rely on them in lieu of a diet restriction. This gives the clearest indication of what benefits may ensue. Even small transgressions will cause a child to "cloud over" or "go back into the fog"—those are phrases parents often share about their children when they consume a wheat or dairy meal again. That said, if giving enzymes with each meal and snack is working in your child's case, go with it. If you are not seeing as much progress as you had hoped for with this method, consider total avoidance of gluten and casein for three months so you can judge the difference.

HELPFUL PROBIOTICS FOR OPIATE-LIKE POLYPEPTIDES

Besides the other benefits they confer for immune function, digestion, and absorption, some strains of probiotic are good at degrading dietary opiate compounds such as gliadomorphin and casomorphin. Two have been reviewed as particularly effective for this so far: *Lactobacillus rhamnosus* and *Lactobacillus crispatus*. Using these strains when a child eats wheat or dairy foods can perhaps mitigate the effects of the opiates. Check labels for inclusion of these strains and look for potencies in the range of 8–10 billion CFUs per dose.

Once you remove gluten, casein, or any other protein source, this is only half the story. *The food you put back in has to be of at least equal nutritional value*, in order for your child to progress. I can't emphasize this enough: Children will usually do poorly on this diet restriction if you give them a poor diet in its place. In fact, it is usually necessary to put food back in that is of *greater* value, to overcome long-term nutrition deficits that were undetected. It is astonishing how often I meet children with autism using a special diet that is inadequate and marginally effective, because the foods put back in are not what the child needs. More on this essential topic in Chapter 4.

Toxicity Testing and Replenishing Micronutrients

After optimizing bowel flora and food intake, and replacing the foods found to be inflammatory or opiate triggers, it is appropriate to look at toxicity issues. Targeted use of supplements can help redirect toxicity. The problem is that because they are so easy to buy and try, many families make the mistake of tinkering with these first. Doing this first will backfire in children who are languishing on poor diets, struggling against inflammation, or buried under organic acids from disruptive bowel flora. If you've tried the infamous high-dose pyridoxine (vitamin B6) and didn't see the heavens open, take heart. It is rare for a single supplement or any single measure to completely redirect a child with multiple nutrition, growth, developmental, behavioral, or learning issues.

This is where some of the more esoteric lab work may come into play. Micronutrients are vitamins and minerals, the essential tiny nutrients we need to run metabolic machinery of every stripe, and to help fabricate tissues and structures in the body. Several of these seem to be out of pace in developmental, psychiatric, and learning diagnoses. Why? Toxic exposures, impaired absorption, inherited disorders of metabolism, and dietary deficits are the culprits for children with autism. Prioritizing what to get at first is made clearer by following the sequence described in this book. If a child is in good growth status, is eating a diet that is supportive of optimal functioning (total calories are adequate; protein, fats, and carbs are adequate for the child's growth status; and appropriate, easily absorbed, noninflammatory sources of macronutrients are used), and bowel flora are supportive of good digestion and absorption, then you can move on to cellular chemistry, and tease apart how to restore broken metabolic pathways. Tests discussed in detail below are those that seem to most confuse parents and providers new to biomedical and diet tools for developmental, learning, and behavioral diagnoses. For any test recommended, be sure your provider explains the treatment path to consider in light of its results.

Urine Organic Acid Test ("OAT")

What it is: A urine test that screens for several organic acids and metabolites that shift, relative to the availability of vitamins and minerals in the body, and relative to the presence of certain toxins.

When to use it: Before any supplements are given, to help guide the protocol; after a long stretch on a supplement protocol, to troubleshoot which nutrients may not be entering the metabolic pathways that need them.

This is a versatile profile that reviews levels of a few dozen metabolic acids in urine that demonstrate the uptake of vitamins and minerals into the pathways where they are needed. When vitamins or minerals are unavailable for their intended jobs (because of poor diet or poor absorption), or if they are somehow blocked from typical distribution into cells (from toxicity or inherited disorders), it is akin to throwing a wrench in the works. Metabolic machinery seizes up; some metabolic chemicals will pile up, others won't get formed at all, and the body will compensate in countless ways, making the need for some nutrients higher. Many of these metabolic goof-ups can be measured in urine with an OAT panel. OAT panels do not measure vitamin and mineral levels directly, but measure levels of organic acids influenced by uptake of vitamins, minerals, and metabolites into cells. This gives clinicians a broad, indirect snapshot of which pathways might need restoration, and how to go about it. Because a urine OAT does not measure levels of vitamins or minerals themselves, a direct serum level of a given micronutrient is necessary in some instances.

Toxic Metals Testing

What it is: A means to check for lead, mercury, antimony, or other toxic heavy metals.

When to use it: If your child was born before 2003 and received the typical vaccination schedule; if your child has received flu shots; if you suspect heavy metal exposures from fish or industrial pollutants; if you live near a coal-burning power plant; if your job exposes you to metals or if you often work with batteries, photographic equipment and film processing, agricultural or industrial chemicals, etc.

This tests for dangerous metals such as lead, mercury, cadmium, and arsenic. These are heavy metals, known to be neurotoxic and poisonous, with long histories of interfering with learning, cognition, normal cellular metabolism, and nerve cell growth. Labs use hair samples, blood, urine, or stool to look for heavy metals. There is a time and place for each of the different methods of looking for these metals. Hair will only reflect an exposure that happened in recent weeks, and was efficiently excreted. A number of studies have demonstrated that children with autism do not show heavy metals in hair. The first trial that looked at this surprised everyone. Carefully matched samples of hair from first baby haircuts were compared for typical children and children who later received autism diagnoses. The typical children's hair had high levels of mercury. The hair from children with autism showed little or none. This was the reverse of what was expected, but it showed that typically developing children excrete the mercury in hair (and ostensibly in stool and urine as well) while children with autism do not. This led to further exploration of the hypothesis that children with autism retain the heavy metal exposures rather than excrete them, and that this is enough mercury to trigger neurological disorders. Mercury has been known as a potent neurotoxin for decades; this is not controversial. The controversial part has become regarding vaccines as a source of mercury big enough to pitch susceptible children into autism or other disorders for speech, learning, attention, or sensorimotor issues. It appears that, for susceptible children, the heavier the exposure, the more serious the diagnosis.

Since the first baby haircut study was published in 2003, other subsequent studies have corroborated that mercury may be retained, not excreted, in kids with autism. Still others have refined the hypothesis that children with autism have a genetic susceptibility to impaired detoxification, meaning that they likely do not excrete mercury well. But the controversy continues, which is why most mainstream pediatricians won't go near this testing for your child with a ten-foot pole! Of course, the real reason is because it hinges on vaccines as a source of mercury. In 2001, the National Institute of Medicine (IOM) stated that a causal connection between mercury in vaccines and autism was "biologically plausible." Then, in 2004, the IOM reversed its position, some say under political pressure, and rejected this hypothesis, even though they ordered a reduction of mercury in children's vaccines. That was too late for children born between 1990 and 2003, who set a precedent by receiving unusually high per-pound doses of mercury as young infants, simply by following the vaccination schedule, which was expanded at that time. One analysis that used the government's Vaccine Safety DataLink data found that infants who received at least 62 micrograms of mercury by three months of age were two and a half times more likely to develop autism. Through the 1990s, infants vaccinated on the recommended schedule received more than that. Even Bernadine Healy, MD, the former head of the IOM, recently expressed concern that public health officials have failed the American public by too hastily dismissing the mercury-autism connection.

How do you know if this is a concern in your child's case? Toxic metals such as mercury and lead are encountered in not just vaccines, but industrial pollutants, too, such as coal emissions or industrial cleaning processes. Mercury exposures to humans can also come from fish, dental fillings, agricultural chemicals, and some medications. We all harbor some toxic metals. Regardless of where these came from, has it reached the tipping point for your child? Lab testing can help you find out, though it can be challenging. Hair will not show the toxic metals in children who retain it. Blood will show only current, not past, exposures of mercury. This is because heavy toxic metals don't like aqueous (watery) environments such as blood. Once your child is exposed, these metals quickly migrate to the fatty tissues they prefer, such as kidney, liver, brain, or nerve tissue. Then they stay there, and stay there, and stay there, triggering repetitive metabolic havoc. So blood is not a useful clinical tool for screening for mercury poisoning, unless you are certain the exposure was very recent. A negative finding in blood will not tell you if a mercury exposure from years ago is gone, or parked in brain tissue. Mercury can end up in teeth, so families that have saved baby teeth can use these, if they can find a lab capable of working with that type of sample. At least one study found higher levels of mercury, but not lead and zinc, in the baby teeth of children with autism versus control (typical) children.

Urine and stool tests can find these older exposures, but only when a chelating or provoking agent is given just prior to the sample collection. Without a chelator or provoking agent, urine and stool panels for heavy metals will not give much information. The chelator grabs the metal and forms a nontoxic, water-soluble molecule that can be excreted. Several compounds can pull poisonous lead, mercury, or other metals out of fatty tissue where they are stuck; then the metals can be measured as they are excreted. This must be done with an experienced MD provider, usually in small pulse doses. Since we all harbor these metals to some degree, a large dose of a chelating agent will likely pull some of them out of most anybody. Excreting too much at once can be unsafe. Different chelating agents each have affinities for some metals over others, and can yank out essential nutrient metals such as zinc or calcium, too, so these must be monitored and thoughtfully replenished during the entire chelating process, which can take months. For a helpful discussion of agents that remove toxic metals, see *Changing the Face of Autism*, by Bryan Jepson (2007), or visit www.geocities.com/autism_mercury/faq.htm.

Because I meet so many parents who have been confused about this, I will repeat: *Metals testing without a provoking agent is not going to measure your child's past exposures to mercury.* Work with a licensed provider who is knowledgeable about this, not new to it, and who explains how your child's essential mineral levels (zinc, calcium, selenium, chromium, potassium, etc.) will be monitored during chelation. Find a provider who has worked with many children successfully in the past. Chelators can have side effects as well, and it is important to know what is typical and safe, and what is unsafe, as your child goes through this often challenging detoxification process. During chelation, it is also important to support pathways that manage detoxification. Per emerging data on children with autism, these pathways (transsulfuration and methylation) are genetically tender to begin with and are likely already disabled before chelation begins. See below for lab tests that some providers use to monitor these detoxification pathways.

URINE PORPHYRIN TEST

What it is: A simple urine test that screens for likelihood of heavy metals toxicity.

When to use it: Before a chelation protocol is begun, a high degree of suspicion that toxic heavy metals are present should be confirmed. This test, plus signs and symptoms, can do that.

An easy way to screen for whether toxic metals burden is an issue for a child is to do a simple test called urine porphyrin. This is a relatively new way to look for heavy metal excess that, so far, has stood up well in a handful of studies. One showed that as urine coproporphyrin levels rose, so did the severity of autism. No provoking agents are needed because this test does not check levels of metals directly, but checks porphyrin pathways disrupted by heavy metal toxicity. If a child's result falls above the reference range for any of the porphyrins screened, further review is probably a good idea. The next step is to talk with your provider about a metals challenge in which your child is given a provoking agent, and you measure metals in urine or stool. I would consider a porphyrin result suspicious if it is high but within the reference range. In this case, carefully review with your provider other signs, symptoms, or lab data to help define the toxicity question.

SPECIAL CIRCUMSTANCES: COPPER IMBALANCE TESTS

What it is: Tests for ceruloplasmin, serum copper, and copper to zinc ratio.
When to use it: When signs of copper excess are present, and you need to confirm treatment protocol with chelation or supplemental minerals.

Copper and zinc were first explored relative to diagnoses such as schizophrenia in the 1960s. These are minerals we must ingest in diets, and they compete for absorption in the gut. In autism, children frequently show copper excess and very low zinc levels. Why, and what does this mean? A leaky gut, which treatment-naive children with autism often have, will allow too much copper to be absorbed. Meanwhile, not enough zinc may be absorbed. Yet another long biochemistry discourse could ensue here, and if you'd like to study up on it, look into metallothionein chemistry for starters (see "Resources and Further Reading"). Essentially, high copper and low zinc levels impede a mechanism to trap toxic heavy metals and push them out of the body. Metallothionein is a ball-shaped cage of a protein that can do that, as long as there is ample zinc around for it to form. Low zinc will also impair immune function, delay growth and sexual maturation, diminish appetite, and slow wound healing. Owing to poor diets, poor absorption, or leaky gut, many kids with special needs don't have nearly enough zinc on board, and may absorb too much copper from the gut.

Copper can become toxic, or even fatal, when it circulates in its unbound form. Signs of this can include tremors, difficulty speaking or swallowing, involuntary jerky movements, or gold-green rings at the cornea of the eye. Hyperactivity, irritability, depression, anxiety, panic attacks, grandiosity, paranoia, phobias, or poor sleep have been noted with excess copper also. Studies from the 1970s showed that supplementing zinc at very high doses with vitamin B6 improved symptoms dramatically for persons with schizophrenia.

If your child struggles with these psychiatric challenges, ruling out a copper imbalance may be a simple measure that could yield a highly effective treatment alternative to Risperdal or other medications commonly given to children. Ceruloplasmin, which is the protein that binds to copper for distribution via blood, is a good place to start. Normally, ceruloplasmin will rise with copper excess.* Though copper doesn't like to travel in blood unbound to a protein such as ceruloplasmin, high levels of unbound serum copper need treatment also to avoid irreversible damage to tissues. Like other metals, it tends to migrate to brain or liver tissue. Supplementing other minerals is usually needed to help excess copper leave the body (zinc, molybdenum, or manganese), and chelating agents are sometimes indicated, too. Looking at the copper to zinc ratio in blood is informative for guiding supplementation, but children can safely use 15–30 milligrams of zinc daily. Some providers use 1 milligram of zinc per kilogram of body weight. Clinical signs for poor zinc status and for copper excess can guide a baseline supplement protocol. Talk with your provider if you suspect more mineral supplementation is needed. As with many lab tests, a chronically poor diet will confound this one, by lowering ceruloplasmin levels.

---

*A genetic disorder called Wilson's disease prevents ceruloplasmin production, even when copper exposure rises.

Supplements for children with autism spectrum issues often exclude copper for the reasons discussed here. Extremely small amounts are adequate and this is likely one mineral your child does not need to supplement if he has autism. Good sources of copper are sesame seeds, tahini, many beans, chickpeas, hummus, soybeans (boiled edamame), sunflower seeds, kale, asparagus, dark leafy greens, cashews, and walnuts. If your child regularly eats something from that list, you may not need to supplement it. Anemia can develop with copper deficiency, and this is easy to rule out with your pediatrician if you are concerned.

OTHER TOXICITY ISSUES: PLASMA CYSTEINE AND PLASMA METHIONINE TESTS

What they are: These are blood tests that tell how well your child's methylation and transsulfuration pathways are working, two major routes for detoxification that are typically problematic in autism spectrum disorders, and possibly in ADHD.

When to use them: This testing may help indicate whether your child will be a responder to methylcobalamin therapy. After bowel flora and diet are optimized is probably the best time to approach this.

Discuss ahead of a detoxification plan when these tests are most informative, since you will want to minimize cost and trauma of blood draws for your child. This is undoubtedly a necessary piece for a clinical trial (in order to clearly demonstrate before and after effects of a supplement protocol), but you can customize, prioritize, and organize this any way you and your provider agree to. In practice, these lab studies can help sort out which children might respond to an inhaled or injected methylcobalamin (methyl-B12) supplement, an excellent tool to restore functioning of these pathways. Since most children with autism show deficits in these pathways, and since this vitamin is very safe to use in high doses, some providers espouse simply starting a methylcobalamin protocol and observing effects. One approach is to obtain this lab data at the beginning for a baseline value, and then perhaps again much later, if the protocol has not triggered a visible benefit.

Some children need folinic (not folic) acid supplemented with methylcobalamin and some do not, and this is where a test for homocysteine and glutathione levels may inform. Homocysteine will be too high when folate status is poor, but depressed in children with inflammation, malabsorption, or toxic burdens. This chemistry gets complicated; some parents like to follow it and some don't. No matter which camp you're in, have your provider offer whatever explanations you need to feel confident in the care plan. See the resources section for information on this topic. Other providers simply like to begin the treatment protocol and add folacin if clinical signs indicate it. If benefits have emerged and your child is showing good progress, then you probably do not need more lab data to continue. Your child is the best indicator of what is going on. Remember, if any specialized measure such as methyl-B12 shots is not working when diagnostic lab work suggested it should, go back to square one and make sure your child's diet is adequate. If it is not, this will impede other treatment measures.

CONVENTIONAL BLOOD TESTS FOR VITAMIN B12 AND ANEMIA

What they are: Complete blood count (CBC), tests for serum folate, serum B12, and methylmalonic acid, and review of red blood cell morphology (shape and appearance).

When to use them: When pernicious anemia must be ruled out.

Historically, the only reason that clinicians have been concerned with vitamin B12 (also called cobalamin) is because it is needed to form normal, iron-toting red blood cells. These tests screen for a distinct form of anemia called megaloblastic (pernicious) anemia, which is caused by poor B12 and folate status secondary to poor diet and malabsorption. These tests are not informative for the methylation and transsulfuration problems now being noticed in autism spectrum and attention deficit disorders. Many clinicians are confused when these conventional blood tests show normal-looking red blood cells and very elevated serum levels of vitamin B12 in children with autism spectrum features, and these are common findings. A compound called methylmalonic acid (MMA) may also be elevated in urine or blood when B12 status is poor. In autism, MMA is often elevated, too.

The problem is that none of these tests gives clear diagnostic information about exactly which form of B12 is problematic in a child with autism, or which form will be therapeutic. B12 occurs in foods, supplements, and in the body in several different forms. It's the methylated form that is frequently thought (though not always) therapeutically relevant in autism spectrum disorders. Ordinary kids' vitamins provide the "cyano" form of B12, which does not treat pathways needing replenishment in autism. There are yet other forms of vitamin B12, too, and providers working with this very hopeful piece of the autism puzzle should be well versed in discerning which form to use. Giving methyl-B12 by mouth does not show the same therapeutic impact as using nasal spray or intramuscularly injected forms that bypass obstacles to absorption in the intestine. B12 is unique in that it needs a specific chemical factor, called instrinsic factor, to cross the intestine and be absorbed into tissues. People with inflammatory bowel diseases may not have this fully on board, and this is why injected or inhaled B12 is of interest. A sequential trial with this tool is emerging as a viable measure for children with autism, who may need ongoing treatment with methyl-B12. Research is new on this tool, but promising. Parents interested in discussing this protocol with their provider can find it outlined, in exhaustive detail, at www.DrNeubrander.com.

Cholesterol Testing in Autism

What it is: Tests for total serum cholesterol.
When to use it: Clinical value for autism remains to be seen.

News that children with autism have unusually low cholesterol levels emerged in early 2008. This was based on a single study that checked a small number of children with autism for a genetic defect known to inhibit cholesterol production. Suddenly everyone was chatting about this test and supplementing cholesterol, even though not a single child in the study was found to have the genetic defect. What they did have was unusually low total cholesterol levels, lower than is healthy. Contrary to what you might think, cholesterol plays a valuable role in our systems. From it, we fabricate molecules to coat nerve fibers and make brain tissue; it is the base for sex hormones, and has several other jobs in the body. Children in pubertal growth spurts especially need good supplies of healthy fats around, so the liver can make cholesterol from dietary supplies of fats and oils. Not only are humans able to make their own cholesterol from dietary fats and oils, we of course also eat cholesterol itself in animal products such as eggs and fatty meats.

What this study did not report on was the growth status, age, or food intakes of the children in the study. Children with a body mass index that is too low, weight too low for height, poor intakes of fats and oils, or poor absorption will all be likely candidates for low total cholesterol levels. These four problems are, as described in the first chapter, typical for kids on the spectrum. There is little point to looking at this for an underweight child—total cholesterol can be low secondary to growth problems and nutrition status, not a genetic defect. Total cholesterol will also dip downward during those big bang growth spurts during puberty, then rebound later when growth velocity tempers itself. If your child has low body mass index, low weight for age, low weight for height, or is about age twelve and growing taller by the hour, you can expect total cholesterol to be low—this is normal for these growth parameters. You can skip the blood test. Restore your child's growth pattern with an adequate diet if it is compromised, and support your budding teen with loads of food and ample healthful fats and oils, if she is skinny and active. You can check total cholesterol then if you like, to see if all is well.

Testing total cholesterol level does not inform on the genetic defect; this is a different test that is not widely available. The treatment for the genetic defect is to use cholesterol itself as a dietary supplement, or eat eggs if they are tolerated. The treatment for low cholesterol in children is to eat adequate total calories and adequate total fats from healthful sources.

TESTING FOR FATTY ACIDS

What it is: Fatty acid blood spot analysis, tests for arachadonic to EPA ratio and triene to tetraene ratio, and individual fatty acid testing for linoleic acid, gamma linolenic acid, and arachadonic acid.

When to use it: If you need to confirm exactly which fatty acid to supplement, or if you have tried fish oil supplementation for several months with no improvement.

Using supplemental oils from flax, fish, borage, evening primrose, black currant, and cod liver is generally safe and healthful, as long as fresh, reputable products are used. Each source has different amounts of the various omega-3 and omega-6 fatty acids; their therapeutic benefits are condition-specific. As mentioned in Chapter 2, children with attention and focus challenges have shown some benefit from docohexasanoic acid (DHA) in higher amounts, while those with mood swings, bipolar disorder, or behavioral volatility seem to need eicosapentanoic acid (EPA) in higher amounts. Others with rough skin and colorless bumpy rashes may benefit from evening primrose oil over other sources. If you have used oils in the amounts described in Chapter 2 for eight to twelve weeks and see no change, there are lab tests that can profile fatty acids, so you can supplement more effectively. Some providers use these before treatment with dietary fish oil supplements. Some base the supplement plan on your child's signs and symptoms.

These oils can trigger improvements in many cases, so if absolutely nothing changes after four months, it might be wise to consider a lab test. I tend to work with a child's presentation for signs, symptoms, and food/supplement intakes rather than lab data to plan doses and sources of supplemental oils—because it usually works well. These clinical signs and symptoms are consistent with compromised status for fatty acids:

- Skin rashes, dry scaly skin, dermatitis
- Decreased skin pigmentation
- Chronic inflammatory conditions
- Chronically watery, greasy, oily, or pale stool
- Mood swings
- Inattention (DHA)
- Hostile or aggressive behavior, tantrums (EPA)

When problems related to fatty acids persist even with supplementation, a lab test can be helpful, as is reviewing fat absorption in the gut. Poor fat digestion and absorption will be obvious in stools as described above, in slowed growth, or in cystic fibrosis; this can result from true pancreatic insufficiency, a condition your gastroenterologist would rule out. Several prescription enzyme preparations exist to help this. More typically, children show ratios of fatty acids in lab tests that reflect their dietary intakes. Most of the time, these ratios are less than ideal to support good focus, attention, or mood. This is where the lab study may help you refine your supplementation protocol, but it is by no means necessary for you to test before giving these oils to your child. Other points to consider:

- Arachadonic to EPA ratio helps confirm if more EPA would be beneficial or if your child is absorbing a high dose of EPA he is already taking.
- Triene to tetraene ratio helps confirm a classic nutritional deficiency of essential fatty acids, linolenic acid and linoleic acid.
- Individual tests for omega-6 fatty acids such as linoleic acid, gamma-linoleic acid, and arachadonic acid are available, but are most useful when expressed as ratios to other fatty acids.
- When fats and oils are generally deficient, fat-soluble vitamins will begin to show signs of marginal status, too, because fat is needed in the diet to absorb these. See page 67 for the Nutrition-Focused Physical Exam, if you would like to review this for your child. Fat-soluble vitamins are A, D, E, and K.

Amino Acids Testing

What it is: Blood or urine is used to define circulating levels of amino acids.

When to use it: Though some clinicians rely on this test often, I have not found it terribly useful for creating nutrition care plans, assessing protein status, or directing amino acid supplementation.

These are profiles that can be created using blood or urine as a sample. They measure amino acids, which are the individual building blocks of proteins, neurotransmitters, hormones, structures, and tissues in the body. Biomedical providers often use them to choose which amino acids might be placed in a supplement protocol. Many parents have brought these lab results to me for interpretation, but I do not find them to be a useful tool in practice, for a number of reasons: First, most children I encounter have predictably poor profiles for amino acids, because they have limited diets and malabsorption. I already know that by looking at their food records (which show me amounts and sources of protein typically eaten per day) and clinical signs and symptoms. Second, amino acids in blood will reflect how well you absorbed the amino acid composition of the protein in your last meal, and that's about it. A fasting sample does not reflect dietary intake well, so it will not inform on how to supplement. Some amino acids stay relatively constant when we are fasting, while others fluctuate, and this again does not give me particularly actionable information. Lastly, gut dysbiosis can interfere with absorption of individual amino acids—and this panel will not give me that information either. These profiles can help a metabolic specialist rule out genetic disorders, but they are not necessary for assessing protein status. Protein status is reliably assessed with signs, symptoms, growth data, and food records, or if need be, with some tests available at your local pediatrician's office. What you need to know is how many protein servings your child needs daily, and from what foods. That is easy enough to figure out without drawing blood. A scoop of an essential amino acid mix can round things out if necessary, and many supplement companies make these for children.

NEUROTRANSMITTER TESTING

What it is: Several companies offer neurotransmitter panels that look for neurotransmitters, hormones, or metabolites relating to mood, sleep, attention, and fight-flight response, usually in urine or saliva samples.

When to use it: Clinical relevance remains unclear. May be useful prior to a medication protocol.

For children with mood concerns, anxiety, or obsessive-compulsive disorder, urine panels are now available that profile levels of several neurotransmitters. These are not able to say what is truly going on in synapses between nerve cells in brain tissue, but some providers claim success with them. A supplement protocol is recommended based on the neurotransmitter profile. Children with autism often have elevated blood serotonin levels, but low levels in the brain; supplementing amino acids that are serotonin precursors can help or hurt the situation, depending on other factors present for the child. I find it more reliable to work with a child's presentation for food intake, growth data, signs, symptoms, and patterns for mood, sleep, anxiety, and so forth. Specific amino acids can be supportive of much improved functioning, in the context of corrected nutrition status and diet overall, but these need to be used as you would a psychiatric medication: in small doses to begin with, individually rather than mixed, and carefully monitored. Some of the amino acids showing promise in this context for children are 5-hydroxytryptophan, N-acetyl cysteine, taurine, carnosine, and theanine. Gamma-aminobutyric acid, or GABA, is sometimes beneficial in large doses but this is not well absorbed from the intestine and hence may not reach cells where it is needed most. Most of these need supportive cofactor vitamins and minerals, which are best assessed and dosed with professional guidance; again, your child's diet must be adequate overall as well.

INTESTINAL PERMEABILITY TESTING

What it is: Testing for serum lactulose and serum mannitol; urine testing may also be available.

When to use it: When you need to monitor the degree of intestinal permeability, as in celiac disease.

Signs and symptoms of intestinal permeability are obvious in infants and children, and treatment for it can begin without specific lab data such as serum lactulose and serum mannitol. So this test may be regarded as an add-on or useful in situations where you need to confirm whether or not measures you have been using have improved intestinal permeability. Signs of intestinal permeability: history of candidiasis (yeast overgrowth) or disruptive bowel bacteria; mixed irritable stools/constipation; food allergies or sensitivities; mood disorders; anemia or vitamin and mineral deficiencies in the context of an adequate diet.

ANTI-STREPTOLYSIN-O (ASO) TITER, VIRAL TITERS

What they are: ASO checks for antibodies to streptococcal infection; viral titers check for antibodies to viruses.

When to use them: When other measures have failed, consider treatment for viral overload. Titers need to be assessed ahead of this to define treatment. ASO titer is assessed when Pediatric Autoimmune Neuropsychiatric Disorders Associated with Strep (PANDAS) are suspected.

PANDAS is a condition that can emerge following a strep throat infection. Essentially, antibodies are made by the body to fight the streptococcal bacteria, but an autoimmune response develops, and the antibodies begin attacking brain tissue. Signs of this would include tics, such as blinking, shoulder shrugging, throat clearing, grunting, or repeating words, that emerge following the resolution of a strep throat infection. Also common are obsessive-compulsive behaviors, oppositional behavior, anxiety, and cognitive inflexibility. If features like these emerge and persist after your child had a strep throat infection that occurred more than six months ago, an ASO titer may help identify the problem. Kids vary with how long antibodies to strep bacteria will circulate after an infection, but if the titer is unusually high and the infection was long ago, this is suspect. Antibiotics are not a promising treatment for PANDAS, since it is autoantibodies, not bacteria, that are the problem in this condition. Autoimmune problems can be helped by nutrition, naturopathic, and homeopathic supports, and sometimes by drugs. Nutrition supports in this situation can include transfer factor, removing inflammatory foods, removing heavy metals like lead or mercury, or replenishing immune supportive nutrients such as zinc, vitamins A and D, or vitamin C.

Wrapping It Up

Many options for lab testing exist, more than I've mentioned here. You don't need them all. Use the Nutrition-Focused Physical Exam discussed earlier, to start with signs and symptoms. Make a list of concerns based on this and start there. Find a provider who respects your involvement, concerns, and financial limitations. Work sequentially, beginning with knowing how much food your child needs daily and planning around that; optimizing bowel flora; replacing the troublesome foods with the right alternatives for your child; then targeting the toxicity issues and using supplementation or medications to correct those. Over time, each step will need revisiting and adjusting. Children with deeper developmental and learning challenges may be in this process for years, while others with minor concerns may benefit from brief physiological redirecting.

I am often asked if it is necessary to rerun lab tests after a nutrition care plan and special diet have been in place for a few months. No, it is not. The true test is your child, and how she is doing. Testing should be triggered by signs and symptoms, not by a calendar. (An exception to this is chelation therapy, which usually requires a scheduled series of tests to see what toxic metals are being excreted.) If problems remain unchanged after several weeks or months of treatments and you cannot say why, further testing can help sort out what your next course of action should be. Each provider will have preferences in terms of lab studies, but remember that your opinion and financial limitations figure into this as well. Otherwise, observe your child. If improvements continue, leave him be. If problems persist, ask your provider which way to turn, and troubleshoot using tools like the Nutrition-Focused Physical Exam, signs and symptoms of bowel problems, or the NCPA steps.

When children have used a well-tuned special diet for some time, have chelated heavy metals, and have worked with a knowledgeable clinician on cellular toxicity layers like methylation, progress should be strong, and you should be seeing your child acquire new heights for functioning and learning. When this doesn't happen, and you are certain that the diet and other tools you have been using are adequate, check into viral titers. This is work for a skilled and curious immunologist. Some children with autism have shown unusually high titers to viral illnesses for which they were vaccinated, or other viruses such as human herpes virus or cytomegalovirus. Their immune systems appear to have overreacted, so to speak, and made too much antibody to the virus in the shot; then the antibody levels remain highly elevated in these cases, as though there is fulminant infection when there is none. Novel treatments for correcting immune function in these cases have shown some promise. It's easy to screen for viral titers (antibody levels) with your pediatrician, if they are willing, but treatment should be supported by a physician who has walked this path before. It may involve antiviral drugs, intravenous immunoglobulin therapy, naturopathic antivirals like transfer factor or herbs, and continued special diet measures. Keep seeking answers, and you may find a fit for your child that you never thought possible. There are may stones to turn over and peek under!

FOUR

Best of All Worlds Special Diet

A Kid-Focused Way to Find the Right Diet Plan for Your Child

The previous chapters have mentioned some of the diets in use for autism spectrum disorders and learning/behavior diagnoses, and some of their pitfalls, including the Specific Carbohydrate Diet (SCD), the gluten-free/casein-free diet (GFCF), and yeast control diets such as the Body Ecology Diet (BED). Not to be left out are low-phenol diets such as the Feingold Diet; the low-oxalate diet; or variations on GFCF in which other foods such as soy, corn, and eggs are also avoided. There are books available that focus on each one of these diets, and information abounds on the Internet about them. It's easy to find protocols, recipes, rationales, and strategies for all these diets. Which one is right for your child?

The truth is that there is no singular diet for autism or any of these diagnoses that suits everyone. There *are* children with big, untreated nutrition problems. Their needs can be as varied as there are stars in the sky. Though every diet has its devotees, my opinion after ten years in practice is that the diet that is best for your child is the one you can follow with the least stress, that makes your child healthy, happy, and more functional socially, physically, and academically. What often works best is your own quirky amalgam of all the diets. This is usually arrived upon after a few months in the trenches experimenting with the most basic changes first and moving forward from there.

That said, there are elements that apply most of the time that enhance success. Aside from following a logical sequence for assessing children as described in Chapter 2 and prioritizing their nutritional needs, I am far from alone in repeatedly finding gluten and casein to be problematic foods for children with autism. Parents of children with less nutritionally complex challenges—ADHD or asthma, for example— often identify just one food they really need to avoid, and a couple of simple supplements, in order for the child to feel much better. The population of children I encounter in practice is almost exclusively comprised of children with autism, ADHD, mood disorders severe enough to keep them out of school, growth problems, inflammation issues, or feeding problems. Most of these children end up avoiding gluten, casein, or both for a period of time, based on findings in the assessment process. The foods avoided comprise just one piece of the entire nutrition intervention. Most of these children also need some supplementation to correct long-entrenched inflammation, toxicity, or marginal nutrition status.

As far as additional restrictions for other foods or using more complex diets, the deciding factors must include what a family can reasonably accomplish, and what is most beneficial for the child. Diets that control oxalates and yeast overgrowth have been around a long time, and can be very good for controlling specific symptoms. But they were never originally intended for children. The children I meet who have begun those protocols are almost always in calorie malnutrition that has already impaired growth; some are also in protein malnutrition. If either of these has been present long enough to slow growth, it has definitely impacted your child's cognitive ability, focus, and functioning for even longer. It's time to change your strategy *so that more food can be given to your child.* If your child truly deteriorates with more food, allow bigger servings of any tolerable foods. Add supports that improve absorption or reduce inflammation; your provider may offer specific suggestions. In other words, if the diet improves symptoms at the expense of your child's growth, it is time for a change. When growth is impaired, so are many other functions in the brain for a child. This is not an acceptable trade-off. Add strategies that make the entire package work better.

Perhaps the biggest key to success with a special diet is to honestly assess ahead of time what your level of commitment can be. All parents want the best for their children, but we are also only human, and have to face our limitations. A stressed-out, overwhelmed parent is not going to comply with a child's special diet. When a parent sabotages my efforts just so he or she can find an off-ramp, because the parent is too overwhelmed, frustrated, and confused and unable to admit it, I know I've probably pushed too far. Just as I do for families I encounter, consider your own limits. Consider that as difficult as using a special diet may seem (and most families find it is not as hard as they had feared), the alternative may be much darker, just as it could be if you skirted a necessary treatment for any chronic disease your child has.

All these diets are symptomatic treatments. That is, they are designed to resolve chronic symptoms such as inflammation, malabsorption, food intolerance, growth and nutrition problems, or toxicity. It is rare for a child with autism to have only one of these problems; most have all at once. It is thus unreasonable to expect a single diet measure to address all the nutrition-related features of the autism spectrum. Don't expect a partial nutrition measure to work like a miracle drug. For example, a Feingold Diet that allows wheat and dairy foods would probably not be successful for a child with autism, but it may work wonders for a child with hyperactivity and no other concerns. What doesn't work is to remove every possible trigger food for the child with autism. If your child is clearly intolerant to food colorings and artificial food additives, has autism with low verbal skills, and shows signs of inflammation, you have a lot on your plate. But you don't have to follow a Feingold, GFCF, and soy-free diet. You can begin with gluten and casein first, and use enzymes, supplements, or Epsom salt baths to help your child tolerate phenols, instead of avoiding every colored food on the planet. Start by getting a grasp on the total amount of food that is appropriate for your child, and work backward from there to make meal and snack plans, using the sequence suggested in Chapter 2. See Chapter 6 for more ideas.

Because diets are essentially symptomatic treatments, the goal is to reduce symptoms; in using medical nutrition therapies, this means helping children tolerate as broad a variety of foods as possible, as soon as possible. If a child appears to tolerate a food well, given signs, symptoms, and lab information, I encourage a parent to keep that food in the mix, even if it defies a particular diet strategy. An example of this is using foods allowed on SCD (which you can find at www.SCDiet.org) but not requiring a child to adhere completely to this diet, if he happens to do well with some of the disallowed foods. Though this idea may rattle some true aficionados of SCD, the point is that the more healed the gut, the less restrictive your diet can become. It is a sign of recovery when a child can reintroduce previous trigger foods and suffer no ill effects. It is a sign that the child is not progressing when, year after year, problems with several food items persist unchanged.

There are conditions in which certain food components must simply be eliminated to avoid worsening a disease process. Autism appears to be one of them. As can occur with celiac disease, or with users of SCD who have Crohn's disease, recovery of intestinal health and overall functioning can happen with special diets for autism. Unlike celiacs, the children with autism can occasionally resume eating all restricted foods at a later point in time, and do well. The only children with autism in whom I have seen this happen are those who have had thorough, professionally monitored nutrition protocols and were also chelated for heavy metals. In these children, the process took years. Yes, a child's autism diagnosis can shift, change, lessen, or even leave, when treatment is complete, coordinated among a cooperative team of providers, and persistent.

At first, my editor bristled when I told her I wanted to use the "R" word—recovery—but recovery is my goal for children I treat with nutrition care. It is a reasonable, appropriate goal. Recovery is a very relative term. Expecting a quick resolution of autism features is not realistic. In the late 1990s and early 2000s, a lot of material circulated to mislead parents that GFCF was a relatively sure and quick tool to "cure" autism. Though it was good news that this intervention was beginning to reach more parents, I met many who were, of course, crestfallen that this wasn't true, and more who abandoned good efforts because of unreasonable expectations. In my opinion, many children with autism whom I've met have shown signs of vaccine injury or complications from antibiotics that were administered by a well-meaning health care system. They have multitiered physiological and immune effects from this, and repairing these injuries takes a long time. The earlier the injury, the deeper the hole your child may be in, and the longer the journey out may take. If your child can shift from profound autism to PDD-NOS, from having autism with no expressive language to having expressive language, or from PDD-NOS to ADD and a learning disability but with typical socialization, that is a brilliant recovery that will serve your child his whole life through. It may mean the difference between finishing college or being unable to attend college, completing a vocational study or needing custodial care. If your child leaves the dungeon of profound autism to function entirely typically, with no special accommodations educationally or nutritionally, you are extremely fortunate to have that rare alignment of the planets that gave your child, and you, all the needed resources to make it happen. Before you begin, check what your expectations truly are, and how long you are willing to work to see them through. Using these tools may lessen or avoid a grim outcome for your child as an adult. The sooner you start, the better for your child.

What Works, What Doesn't

Aside from starting off by expecting too much too soon, parents tend to stumble into a number of pitfalls along this special diet path. To avoid a derailment of your valuable efforts, check this list before you start, and consider these alternate suggestions.

Pitfall: Diving in with no plan

Avoid it this way: Create a plan before you start. Identify your wishes and hopes; then identify what you expect will happen, even if it's negative. Being honest with yourself up front works better in the long run. If you fully expect a negative outcome, you may create one. Draft an agreement for yourself, your spouse or adult caregivers who are in this with you, and even your child's primary provider. Identify how long you are willing to work at this, and what you need to see for results in order to continue. Are you willing to do this to improve your child's health and functioning to some degree, or are you only interested in completely vanquishing an autism diagnosis? Many have not been able to achieve this, but have seen large enough shifts to keep going.

Pitfall: Bypassing or delaying the bowel flora piece

Avoid it this way: Treat bowel flora first, or at the same time as starting your child's special diet. Treat it as aggressively as possible to start. You will get a greater positive response sooner. It is common for little progress to be seen on a special diet, even when compliance is good, if disruptive bowel flora are still in there noshing on your child's new foods and supplements, and sending their toxins to your child's brain.

Pitfall: Removing only gluten and casein, and treating nothing else

Avoid it this way: Assess your child's total nutrition needs by following the steps outlined in Chapter 2. Removing these two proteins is not enough to treat all the nutrition problems children with autism have. It can bring initial positive signs, but without a total care plan, your child may soon plateau for improvement. Find a provider you like, support groups, or other families using these tools, and implement the entire process. Many parents tell me, "We tried the diet and it didn't work"—this often means they used an unmonitored, nutritionally inadequate GFCF trial, did not address bowel flora correctly, and randomly tinkered with supplements. *No parent should expect to know how to do medical nutrition therapy correctly without some professional guidance, peer support, or help.*

Pitfall: Waiting for "scientific proof" to justify special diets

Avoid it this way: Start now. The proof we would all like to see may take years, and will probably not arrive in a package that satisfies the American Academy of Pediatrics. Decades of solid science in child nutrition already corroborate therapeutic nutrition care for bowel disease, inflammation, and toxicity. This is not new, not alternative, and not unproven. Putting it together for what have been regarded solely as psychiatric disorders in children is new, but the nutrition tenets underneath are of the same science that has been present for decades. Merging this with new research on toxicity and oxidative stress in autism or ADHD might well be a winning combination for your child.

Pitfall: Using a trial period that is too short (two months or less)

Avoid it this way: Use a longer trial period, at least six months, with all pieces of your total nutrition plan implemented and with as total compliance as you can achieve, before judging any changes.

Pitfall: Expecting too much success too soon for a child with autism

Avoid it this way: See the opening paragraphs of this chapter.

Pitfall: Removing fluid milk only, and not other casein sources

Avoid it this way: Visit www.gfcdiet.com for a list of casein-containing foods that must be withdrawn. Children who continue to eat casein daily will not progress as well as those who avoid all casein. Yogurt, cheese, Goldfish crackers, creamy dressings, cheese on pizza, and sherbet are foods parents often forget to remove.

Pitfall: Replacing fluid milk with rice milk, potato milk, or soy milk

Avoid it this way: Use free amino acid protein sources to replace casein if your child does not eat other proteins such as eggs, meats, fish, or chicken. Beans, quinoa, Quorn, peas, or corn are helpful, too, but do not have a protein quality (amino acid profile) that is high enough to be solely relied upon, and some children either refuse them or can't tolerate these either. Supplemental powders such as AminoPlex work in fruit smoothies, or use formulas such as Splash, which come in a ready-to-feed juice box format. Ultracare for Kids powder works in some cases as well. Milks from rice, potato, almond, hazelnut, and hemp contain little to no protein and are poor for fats. They are mostly simple starch. They make fine milk substitutes for baking or smoothies, but using these as a major daily replacement for dairy will leave your child malnourished. Soy protein is a fair protein source, but is similar to casein in terms of its digestive process. That means that it, too, can elicit opiate-like compounds. Occasional use of soy can work for some kids—it is present as flour in well-liked items such as gluten-free pretzels—but it should not be relied upon as a daily major protein source in fluid soy milk, soy yogurt, or tofu for kids with positive urine polypeptide findings.

Pitfall: Not removing both gluten and casein

Avoid it this way: Remove both. Plan ahead of time which one you find easier to withdraw first. If one is malabsorbed, the other one usually is, too, for children on the autism spectrum. If you withdrew one and saw progress, expect to see more by also withdrawing the other, even if a urine polypeptide analysis did not show opiates from both. Children with ADHD, asthma, or other, less nutritionally complex diagnoses may do well with targeting just one of these, and this can be learned through ELISA. (See Chapter 3.)

Pitfall: Giving in to obstacles, fears, or your child

Avoid it this way: Children with autism spectrum issues, OCD, anxiety, or sensory integration disorder are legendary for being obstinate. Expect obstinacy and you will be more able to overcome it. Once we've begun a special diet or therapeutic nutrition measure, it is common for parents to call me and insist their child is refusing new foods, the antifungal medication, a needed supplement, or is just plain bucking any change demanded of him. Just as you give your child an antibiotic if it is needed, give medications and supplements if they are needed. You want your child's health and functional abilities to be as strong as possible. If you have doubts about the protocol or can't comply with a piece of it, clear the air with your provider, so your confidence can be at its fullest. Your resolve and leadership will benefit your child and set a firm, guiding tone. If your child is not progressing, slowing down for growth, or showing new signs of depression, anxiety, behavior, or mood concerns since beginning a nutrition protocol, tell your provider. You need a new plan that works for your child, and that you can confidently administer. Though initially nutrition care and special diets can trigger an illness or challenging behavior, your child should be progressing toward better growth, appetite, functioning, and learning—not the other way around.

Pitfall: For children with ADHD, concerns for mood, depression, anxiety, focus, or irritability, expecting a gluten-free diet to make sudden and dramatic changes.

Avoid it this way: Stick with the trial period for longer than two weeks. If your child has these concerns and testing shows an elevated antigliadin antibody, it is quite possible that a gluten-free diet can improve things. But your child won't turn the corner as fast as a child with true celiac disease, once gluten is withdrawn. Two weeks is not long enough for benefits to emerge. Gliadin antibodies can remain high for weeks or months after the last gluten exposure, and benefits can ensue only when those antibody levels start to drop. This is also why it is so important not to cheat during the initial trial by serving pizza "only on the weekends." This will completely topple the progress you seek and place you back at square one. Every gluten exposure triggers more gliadin antibody production. Try going gluten-free for at least three months, and ideally even longer, before gauging the changes. Keep a daily log of your child's status with a 1 to 10 rating. For example, if ADHD is the issue, rate your child's behavior daily, with 1 being the worst, 5 being baseline for your child, and 10 being fantastic. If depression and social withdrawal dog your child, create a gauge for this, too, and assign a value to it daily. Include notes on unusual changes. The impact of a gluten-free diet may otherwise be too subtle and gradual for you to appreciate. Keep tabs on growth as well; if growth lunges ahead within the gluten-free trial, this may be confirmation that you're on the right track. If you're still not convinced after a conscientious four-month effort, let your child go eat the pizza, breadsticks, and chocolate cake. If behavior problems ensue in an abrupt, dramatic fashion—tantrums, hyperactivity, diminished ability for social context, poor sleep, or a return of "stim" activities like lining up trains, spinning things, or playing with window blinds—well, now you know! You have probably unleashed opiate-like compounds, inflammatory proteins, or both into your child's body. These will quickly overwhelm a child who is early in the recovery and repair process, and this kind of reaction implies you'd best return to the diet strategy for now.

Pitfall: Starting with supplements

Avoid it this way: Start with food. Get a feel for how much food your child needs daily in terms of calories, and plan out meals working from there. Allow a baseline multivitamin mineral supplement such as Klaire Labs VitaSpectrum powder (easy to dose slowly and easy to give to anyone who can't use capsules—although capsules are available also). Once you have balanced bowel flora and know which replacement foods are on the menu, supplements can be targeted more effectively for specific problems.

Pitfall: Relying solely on IgE allergy testing to define inflammation from foods

Avoid it this way: Use an ELISA with IgG testing panel to get a broader snapshot and help you prioritize foods your child can use. If a picture of overall inflammation is present—that is, a dozen or more highly reactive foods—you will need to work aggressively with gut health supports such as probiotics, antifungals, liposomal glutathione, or n-acetyl-cysteine. Herbs such as aloe, chamomile, slippery elm, ginger root, and marshmallow root can also soothe the GI tract and accelerate healing. Most parents I meet tell me at the outset that their child has already been tested for food allergies, and the findings were negative. Invariably, this means that an IgE RAST test was done, which is incomplete information for our purposes here.

Pitfall: Making meals for your special-needs child separate from the rest of your family (different foods, separate seating, or different mealtimes than family members)

Avoid it this way: Don't impose an extra degree of separation by feeding your special-needs child a different plate of food from other family members. Make family meals that meet your child's diet restrictions, so that he or she can share in the family meal as often as is reasonable, even if it is a routine only one night a week. Four nights a week is even better. Many children with sensory defensiveness cannot stand cooking smells, the noise of tableware, or the sight of others chewing. Just being at the table can be an overwhelming, anxiety-provoking experience for them. This can leave them eating alone most of the time. Others simply can't sit still and need to be up and moving between every bite. If it causes your child more stress than it prevents to join everyone at the table, let her be, but give her the same meal that everyone else is having. Make it obvious that the same foods are given to everyone on a regular basis—so that even if you accommodate your child by letting her eat in a separate spot, she knows she is included in the meal, because she gets to eat what everyone else is eating. This is very important. Several menus are innately workable in a gluten- and/or casein-free diet. For example, if you eat together one night a week, serve hot dogs, French fries, coleslaw, and watermelon—and no one is left out. Not haute cuisine, but everyone is included. Grilled meats and sides of potato, rice, and vegetables always fit this agenda. Families who do this have more success and stick with the intervention longer than families who eat in splinter groups with different foods in front of everyone. It also sends a clear message to your child with special needs that she belongs in the family. While it can fail to force a child with high sensory defensiveness to struggle through a meal seated at the family table when she just can't do it, she can always be included by being given the same foods as parents and siblings, no matter where she sits.

Pitfall: Turning to teachers, family, or the pediatrician for approval before you start

Avoid it this way: Your allies and supports are going to matter a lot as you embark on this journey, so be sure you've picked the right ones. Sometimes the people who should support us don't or can't, and you may have to find others, or move on. If your child's teachers, aunts, grandparents, and doctors already knew what a great idea a special diet is, you would have heard them telling you to do it by now. If they have, great! That's a good place to start for support. Ultimately, though, as the parent, this is your decision, not theirs. If you are resolute in yourself that this is something you want to do for your child, the supports and resources you need will come. Find supporters on email lists or online chat groups; check qualifications and experience of providers you may like to work with; talk to anyone on your provider team who may have ideas; or ask trusted parents of special-needs children like yours. This intervention is new for most pediatricians. If yours is not supportive or willing to learn, find other qualified providers who are.

Pitfall: Needing your child's cooperation to get started

Avoid it this way: Don't expect cheerful compliance, or any compliance, from your child if he has an autism spectrum disorder. Go forward anyway. Perhaps your child did not want to attend his first day of school, get his first shot, begin ABA, take a medicine he needed, or stay with a sitter the other night. You did it anyway. Be resolute and calm. You are in charge. If your child truly can't manage a supplement, ask your provider for an alternative form that might be easier. There are powders, liquids, chewables, oral sprays, nasal sprays, and topical versions of vitamins. As for trying new foods, it can take several weeks for these to be even sniffed at by a child with autism. You simply have to wait for the gluten- and casein-sourced opiate compounds to leave the brain, as these arrest interest in other foods for as long as they are circulating. This takes weeks, and some children will show a diminished food intake in this stretch as they hold out for their old favorites. This is when parents get to see just how addicting these protein fragments are for children on the spectrum! Provide fluids, and plenty of whatever foods your child will accept in this phase even if they are less than optimal. Also allow trades ("After you drink this, we can turn on the TV"), reliable distractions such as soothing Epsom salt baths with some toys and a few drops of calming lavender; grandparent or favorite caregiver visits; bottles (yes, some children with autism use bottles to age four or even six); pacifiers; chewy toys; swings; videos; repeat visits to favorite locales such as the carwash, zoo, pool, hardware store; or whatever distractions you find helpful to pull your child through this hard part of opiate withdrawal. Children may be downright crabby during this phase. It will pass. If it doesn't pass in four to six weeks, holler for your provider to troubleshoot why. Antifungal therapy usually speeds this part up. The longest I have seen this phase last is nine weeks, and that was in a two-year-old child—as young as this is, he made it through, even though he dipped for good total calorie intake for a while. He rapidly progressed after this long and daunting withdrawal, with a course of Diflucan.

Pitfall: Removing every reactive food on an ELISA panel
Avoid it this way: Start with the three top offenders, rotate the others, and add supplements that support gut tissue healing to reverse intestinal permeability: antifungal treatment (as aggressive as can be permitted and tolerated), high-potency probiotics, glutathione (which is not absorbed well beyond the gut, but may help gut tissue itself), and herbs. Removing all of the offending foods is too restrictive for children, unless they are able to use a formula such as Splash, upto 32 ounces per day or more.

Pitfall: "My child only eats wheat and dairy foods, so therefore this diet won't work for him"
Avoid it this way: Yes, it could. This set of food preferences is often a strong and favorable clinical sign that the diet *will* work. Your child is probably addicted to opiate-forming compounds in those foods, and unable to stop eating them without intervention.

Pitfall: Overrestricting carbohydrate intake, fat intake, or total food intake
Avoid it this way: Go back to Step 1: Is your child eating enough total calories? Get a feel for your child's daily needs for total calories,

and allow adjustments as necessary. Check for signs and symptoms of low total calories. Make sure your child is not languishing there. Kids need calories, kids need carbs, and kids need fats and oils. Overrestricting a child's intake is harmful. Children with calorically poor diets in infancy and toddlerhood can suffer persisting cognitive deficits as a result, detectable at age seven years. Early childhood is not the moment to overrestrict calories, protein, fats, or carbohydrates. As was mentioned earlier in Chapter 2, a special diet has probably become inadequate when a child shows an initial great response, only to peter out a few weeks later, with a return of some problem behaviors or a regression of some new skills that popped out at the start. Don't get stuck worrying that the food you add back will do harm. Withholding food does harm. If a measure like SCD or yeast control diets triggered a nice early response, you have some confirmation that yeast is an issue for your child. That's good information. In that case, instead of not feeding your child enough food to grow and think, feed him, and implement strong antifungal therapies and probiotics to counter the yeast. If you tried a low-oxalate diet and saw a stunning first response that fizzled into the same old same old, that is also excellent information. It suggests that oxalates need controlling, but again, it backfires to simply not feed your child enough food, in order to control oxalates. Perhaps your child would benefit from VSL3, a probiotic that degrades oxalates in the intestine, or from more antifungal supports. *Lactobacillus acidophilus* and *Streptococcus thermo* are two probiotic strains that can also degrade oxalates. Adding a cup of baking soda to the cup of Epsom salts in nightly baths can accelerate the removal of irritating oxalates, too. What you can know for sure is that if you don't give your child the food he needs, he will suffer behaviorally, cognitively, functionally, and eventually for growth as well.

Pitfall: Expecting a child to need or accept the same foods an adult needs (low fat, low carb, lots of roughage, fiber, and raw foods)

Avoid it this way: Allow room for typical kid treats. Honor special occasions with a cake, cupcakes, or whatever is appropriate. Special versions abound to accommodate dietary restrictions for wheat, dairy, egg, soy, and so on. This is not to say that raw foods, fermented foods, and fiber are bad for children. It is to say that because they are growing, they need more calorie-dense foods than adults do (up to twice the calories per pound than us grown-ups), and can't exclusively rely on low-calorie, high-fiber, or high-water-content foods. Raw and fermented foods are great, and healthful for everyone. But when used to the exclusion of other foods, they don't provide enough food energy for a growing child.

Pitfall: Avoiding special events because of diet restrictions

Avoid it this way: Rise to the occasion. Cookbooks abound to help you create desserts, mains, sides, breads, rolls, pizza, calzones—whatever—for holidays, birthdays, school parties, or what have you, without offending foods. See the resources section for ideas. SCD users are legendary for creating unusual and delicious desserts—nuts and eggs are often in these recipes, so a caution goes out to children who may have inflammation from those. For years I was the annoying mom who brought a GFCF cake to the birthday party, so that my son could eat cake, too, and share with the other kids. Who doesn't like two cakes? Usually, moms didn't mind and the kids loved having two desserts. I have also made CF eggnog that nobody detected as anything but good, entirely GFCF Thanksgiving meals from soup to nuts, and hosted the dessert portion of a neighborhood progressive dinner, gluten-free (as it happens, I have two gluten-intolerant neighbors, which makes my son feel like one of the gang). Special occasions matter, and it's important for children on diet restrictions to partake of the same special foods as everyone else does.

Pitfall: Telling a young child too much detail about the diet and its purpose
Avoid it this way: Tell your child only what he truly needs to know to continue to feel loved, accepted, and confident. Too much information will create anxiety and confusion for a child. If he asks for information at all, which he may not, use concrete examples from his own life. For example, a child who has struggled with potty training or has painful bowel movements might be able to comprehend that eating different foods may ease this. Your child will then expect the very next BM to be a breeze, so if you can't deliver on your promise, don't make it. Instead say, "After a few days, this may begin to make your BMs easier. If you want to, tell me if you notice your BMs feeling better." Or: "These foods might help you have fewer tummy-aches. Tell me if you notice." For nonverbal children, you obviously can't expect a report on progress, but receptive language is often intact. Use the same simple and direct language you do for anything else, but give only information they truly seem to need. A suitable approach for toddlers is not to give any information at all. Simply begin switching in new foods. When it comes to using supplements, find forms they accept most and make them a routine, like brushing teeth, putting away toys, or learning to say hello. Connect the supplements to a daily ritual so they are easily remembered—like placing them at your child's breakfast table setting in a little cup, or serving it (if it's a liquid) in the same drink every day at breakfast. Some families succeed by putting supplements in soft foods or drinks the child is sure to finish (but this may backfire for older children, who figure out your sneaky tactics). For older and higher-functioning children, the same rule applies: Whatever they inquire about, you can share information in concrete terms. "The testing we did shows that this might make it easier for you to focus at school," or "you might be less bothered by noise or tags if we use

this; it may work slowly, so we can keep track if you like," or "this may help you feel less anxious/sleep better/have more energy . . ."

Pitfall: Relying on hair testing to define which supplements and chelators to use

Avoid it this way: You and your provider can use clinical signs, symptoms, and thoughtfully selected data from urine, stool, or blood to define this important phase of your intervention. Hair testing can have its place, but other tools work as well or better. Hair reflects what happened last week, or longer ago. Nutrient or toxic metal levels in hair do not necessarily have direct linear relationships with levels for these in the body and can thus be misinterpreted.

Pitfall: Giving up when a child refuses a food or supplement

Avoid it this way: Give new items several tries before you give up on them. Studies have shown that typical children refuse a new food as many as twelve times. Guess what children with autism do? They refuse more vehemently and for longer. Expecting this can help you stay neutral. If a child refuses a new item, you can reintroduce it again on another day. If this means your child will miss a meal or snack, allow reliable favorites for calories, and be sure to provide ample fluids—like smoothies, juice without added sugar or corn syrup, water, or specialized formulas you have been instructed to use. Kids need calories and can't go for long stretches on fumes, like adults can. Most children transitioning to GFCF diets will still eat French fries (for better or worse) so if you are very concerned that your child has had no calories on a given day, allow a transgression of a starchy food like this to carry her through. If appetite rigidity persists for more than a few weeks, it is time to troubleshoot, and ask your provider if you are out of ideas. Your child should not be losing weight, so do contact your provider if this is happening. If you have withdrawn only one of the opiate peptide proteins, then withdrawing both may improve things. Make sure bowel flora are tip-top also.

Pick a Strategy: Is This Your Kid?

Rather than focusing on the details of each diet strategy, I like to focus on kids. Here are a few common profiles that tend to come across my office threshold a lot. See if your child fits one of these, and try the suggestions that follow to get you off and running for the first few weeks. After that, you will need input from a qualified provider to optimize supplementation; review toxicity, inflammation, or viral issues; and treat any unexpected obstacles that come up.

THE MILK-ADDICTED KID

These are kids who are still using fluid milk as a major protein and calorie source well past the age of twelve months, when weaning off breast or formula as a major calorie source should be under way. They are drinking 40 to 60 ounces of milk a day (that's about five to eight cups). They are literally addicted to milk—and experiencing a neurotransmitter effect from it that is not typical. Developmentally, children with autism who are milk-addicted seem to show the more profound language delays. When they are on the younger end, say age three or four, they may be almost nonverbal or will have begun speaking late. If they are school age, say six or so, they may have expressive language praxis issues, meaning that they can talk but not in a typical way. They may use echolalic language (repeating what they hear), refer to themselves in the third person, or misunderstand social context. This is often the first area of functioning that shifts when dietary opiates begin to disengage: Your child may begin to use language in a new, more typical way; make eye contact; or comply more typically with your requests. So removing dairy can be very successful.

When milk is a big calorie source in children over one year, it displaces solid calories and reduces intake of other foods they very much need at this age and stage. They refuse other foods and have oral tactile defensive issues, meaning they refuse varied textures in foods, hate to eat or chew, perhaps have delayed chewing skills (which is why some stick to the bottle in the first place), or rely on suckling to calm themselves neurologically. Since oral tactile issues are common in autism spectrum disorders and sensory integration disorder, it's not unusual for these children to drink from a bottle beyond age three. When they accept foods, it is often dairy items that they choose—sweet yogurt, cheese, ice cream. A few random solids might be in the diet, but on balance, their diets lack most essential minerals, some vitamins, appropriate fats, and sometimes, total calories. There is often pallor, allergic shiners, white dots on fingernails, and a blank countenance. Parents in this predicament sometimes turn to high-calorie milk-based drinks such as Peptamen Junior, Carnation Instant Breakfast, or Boost, hoping to provide a few micronutrients and extra calories. This won't work. It leaves the child addicted to opiates formed from casein, the protein source in these drinks.

These are children with neurological and sensory challenges, not bad parents. Withdrawing the milk, and the bottle if there is still one in the picture, can work, if appropriate replacements are provided. If not, your efforts may simply backfire, entrenching your child's dependence on the bottle or milk, and fear of losing these, even more deeply. You need a nutritious milk replacement, mineral replenishment, bowel flora correction, and a sensory integration plan to replace the neurological organization that sucking on the bottle gives the child.

WHAT TO DO: Talk to your child's occupational therapist, if you have one, about what can replace the bottle in terms of its neurological benefit. Children with sensory integration disorder using a bottle at a late age may legitimately need this oral activity for self-calming, which they might not have mastered in other ways. Suddenly removing it with no alternative may trigger more setback than progress. For example, a few inches of surgical tubing can be knotted for a child to suck, chew, and pull.

■   ■   ■

As for nutrition, replace any gluten foods in this child's diet first. Since these are not the opiate of choice for this child, it usually won't be noticed that the cookies, pasta, bagels, microwave macaroni and cheese, and frozen pizza are going gluten-free. Swap in the gluten-free versions with zero fanfare—and zero information, unless your child is old enough and functional enough to ask a few questions. Age of readiness for this will vary with each child's level of expressive language and functional ability, so trust your instincts here, and err on the side of giving too little information. If your child needs more info and can ask for it, he probably will.

Successfully launch that transition first, and save yourself for the much bigger battle: withdrawing casein. Before you begin this, take care of bowel flora as aggressively and completely as possible, and begin nightly Epsom salt baths if possible, to replenish magnesium and sulfur. You may begin introducing casein-free ingredients where they won't be noticed at first. For example, if the child likes pancakes, use one of the many gluten-free pancake mixes* now available, and instead of using cow's milk to mix the batter, use almond milk. For cupcakes and treats, use GF mixes, almond milk, and Earth Balance margarine instead of butter. Yes, you do have to withdraw butter, because it has milk protein solids in it, as does any margarine with casein ingredients. Gradually offer more and more favorite solid foods, and offer them before liquid nourishment, which fills the stomach with more volume than calories. Next, add minerals—especially zinc. Try VitaSpectrum Powder in applesauce or capsules if they can be swallowed. Give zinc, up to 30 milligrams per day, for the first two weeks to trigger appetite and replenish what has been lacking for a long time. This is available in many forms, from colorless liquid to flavored liquid to chewables. Then, the big moment: Eliminate the milk. In its place, use Splash formula, Neocate One Plus, Pepdite, smoothies made with Ultracare for Kids or AminoPlex—whatever your child will take. After about a week,

---

*Of these, while a brand called Pamela's is delicious, it has buttermilk in it, which is disallowed on a casein-restricted diet.

expect fireworks, and hunker down. This is when the opiates will begin to vacate endorphin receptors and your child may start to be very unhappy with this new plan. Don't crack now. Mineral replenishment, tackling gluten first, and cleaning up the bowel flora ahead of time will make this stage go more quickly and with less trouble.

The Yellow Diet Kid

Mac and cheese. Cheese pizza. SpaghettiOs. Goldfish crackers, Cheez-It crackers, Ritz crackers. Pancakes. Belgian waffles. Doughnuts. French fries. Bread. Bread. Did I mention bread? (One toddler I met would literally bore through the middle of a long loaf of soft white bread daily like a drill, leaving the crusts. Nothing else, just bread.) Fast-food burgers or chicken nuggets. Did I miss anything? These are children hooked on starchy wheat calories, but they hate milk and don't drink it. Juice? No problem. Gluten is often the polypeptide that is elevated while casein may be in range.

WHAT TO DO: As always, begin with a calorie range you know will suit your child, followed by bowel flora corrections. Then, do the reverse of what is done for milk-addicted children: Replace the casein first. Begin by putting a high-nutrient substitute for juice in the mix, since this child usually likes juice. It will be needed when the starchy wheat is withdrawn and the child starts refusing to eat. Use one of the free amino acid options I keep mentioning: Splash, Odwalla juice drinks with AminoPlex powder, Pepdite, or your own concoction. These should have at least a gram of protein per ounce (so an 8-ounce drink should have 7–8 grams of protein) and 150 calories or more per 8 ounces. If you really need to boost calories, add unsweetened coconut milk. Give two of these drinks daily (16 grams of protein), three if your child won't touch meats, fish, or chicken. Next begin sneaking in the gluten-free versions of everything "yellow": Bell & Evans gluten-free chicken nuggets or tenders, in the freezer section at better supermarkets; Van's gluten-free frozen waffles, or make your own in the waffle iron with a GF mix; Tinkyada brand GF pastas (my personal favorite). Buy GF bread from Kinnikinnick or Whole Foods (check for milk ingredients) and use it to make French toast for breakfast. Pasta for lunch, gluten-free. Instead of mac and cheese, which is truly a challenge to mimic without good real cheese, try GF macaroni elbows with olive oil or Earth Balance Margarine (not butter), garlic salt, and pepper. No Parmesan (that's cheese, too). The multi, zinc, bowel flora fix, and Epsom salts ought to all be on board before or during the gluten removal, to ease withdrawal symptoms.

THE SUDDEN VEGETARIAN

What is it about prepubertal Asperger's boys that makes them do this? I have a cluster of clients whose Asperger's sons randomly and emphatically decided around age ten that they were vegetarian. A vegetarian diet can be challenging for an entirely typical child to grow on, but for a child needing to restrict wheat, dairy, and soy foods, it is exceptionally hard. These children usually begin at low weight for height, low BMI, or some slowed growth velocity already—so eating even less high-quality protein is the last thing they need. But it can be done. Since Asperger's can feature obstinacy or cognitive rigidity, it can make sense to let this child gain some sense of control and empowerment by permitting this junket. Make a contract with this child that you are willing to permit it for four to six months. If the child's growth has shown a downward shift, which you can identify using percent ideal body weight or body mass index, then the rule is he must return to eating animal or fish protein sources, and more calories.

WHAT TO DO: Rotate alternative high biological value protein sources such as Quorn, the amino acid–based formulas and powders, eggs, and fish, if the child will allow it. Complementing lower-value protein sources, as any vegetarian is accustomed to doing, is necessary. This means serving beans with rice or corn, so that their amino acid profiles complement each other to form higher-value protein. The protein in beans and whole grain brown rice is harder to extract, because of the fiber content of these foods. If your child is struggling with gas, add enzymes and probiotics to the routine. While tofu, soy yogurt, and soy milk are fine for vegetarian diets, these are not ideal for daily use in Asperger's or autism spectrum disorders, owing to their propensity to form an opiate-like compound. If the child has no intolerance or allergy to soy, using it occasionally may work, but you will need to watch for tolerance. As always, supplements need to thoroughly address minerals such as zinc, selenium, and possibly iron, as well as the full complement B group. Make sure fats are adequate, to support typical prepuberty and pubertal growth spurts. Use unsweetened coconut milk to create thick creamy smoothies as a base for amino acid powder; add flavors your child likes—vanilla, almond, pineapple, banana. Stick to the contract. If your child has shown a clear growth regression on this diet, discuss relaxing the vegetarian restriction. Add ample fats and carbohydrates, and insist on high-value protein daily.

THE REFLUX KID

These are children who got off on the wrong foot from day one. Typically, there was a neonatal situation that meant bowel flora was never imprinted properly on the child's gut and immune system: a C-section delivery, early or repeated antibiotics in the first weeks, using whole cow's milk formula in a less than 40-week-old gestational age infant, or giving a breast-feeding mom an MMR shot or booster right after delivery (thus dosing the baby with viral material via milk at birth). A merry-go-round of illnesses, growth problems, and developmental quirks or delays often ensue. The baby often cannot tolerate even breast milk, and attempts at various formulas come next. Part of the story is that nothing was ever normally tolerated in the baby's gut. Reflux appears early and persists; first, Mylicon drops are given to no avail, then it's on to stronger prescriptions for reflux. Medications that are meant to be used for a few weeks at most become long-term crutches for the child, used indefinitely. Candidiasis becomes an entrenched nightmare. Allergy testing is done (IgE), but of course, it's inconclusive and incomplete, and IgG testing is usually overlooked. The child's appetite is extremely picky, with a penchant for yellow diet foods. There is oral tactile defensiveness to a degree that parents may have to put food in the child's mouth well past age three, because the child hates to do it. Herculean distractions are needed to get the food in: videos, stories, anything to pull the child's attention away from food going in the mouth. Growth lags. Developmentally, children with autism stuck in the reflux loop seem to show a kind of fractured pattern, with fits and starts. Like most kids on the spectrum, they are extremely bright, but behavioral and cognitive rigidity is deep.

WHAT TO DO: Reboot the bowel flora. It never got situated in the first place, and this set off the downward spiral of intolerance and sensitivities, allergy, and reflux. If this child is using a medication such as Prevacid, and strong antifungal medication is contraindicated, use Nystatin at the highest allowable dose for four to six weeks; discuss dosing with your doctor. This is challenging, because Nystatin must be given three to four times per day, but it may be worthwhile to redirect all the GI issues present in this case. Nystatin is safe to use for long periods, over a month if necessary. If a stronger, systemically acting azole antifungal medication is not contraindicated by use of other prescriptions your child needs daily, use it. It's easier (once-a-day dosing) and it has a farther reach in the body (Nystatin acts only in the gut). Toward the second half of antifungal treatment, bring in a probiotic. Which is best is hard to say. If you were able to get a stool culture first, base your probiotic choice on beneficial strains that were already successfully growing

in the sample, and try boosting those (see Chapter 3 for details). If nothing beneficial was growing, you could try starting with the very first flora
that never got there in the first place: Bifidobacterium species (*B. breve*,
B. infantis, *B. lactis*, *B. longum*) and certain Lactobacillus strains that
appear early to support the human infant's gut (*L. casei* and *L. rhamnosus*). Dose these high, at least 10 billion CFUs per day. In practice, I
prefer Klaire Labs' products for this job. It is unclear if children over one
year can benefit from these strains or not, but I have found that when
strains that typically populate the gut of a healthy older child are supplemented in reflux kids, they sometimes don't take. It's as though the
sequence has to go back to square one and start itself where it was
meant to. Experiment with different probiotic blends and strains to see
what works best for your child.

Pulling a kid out of the reflux loop is hard and may take months.
Reflux medication is shortsighted. It changes stomach acid pH so that
what is refluxed into the esophagus is less irritating. This is a good
short-term answer. Over the long run, though, keeping stomach pH too
alkaline (rather than very acidic, as it is meant to be) will keep food in
the stomach longer, which will increase the likelihood of it refluxing
back into the esophagus. Thus, reflux kids tend to need higher and
higher doses of this medication. They reflux more, increase the dose,
and reflux even more. Eventually, the pH of the entire GI tract can
shift. Even small pH shifts will change what bowel flora thrive in there.
A more alkaline environment favors yeast overgrowth, and the cycle of
dependence on medication worsens even more. The goal is to correct
the bowel flora so that it aids digestion, then gently and gradually normalize stomach acid so that digestion can begin normally in the stomach and the pH of the digestive tract can support healthy flora.

Wean your child off reflux medication slowly with permission from
your doctor. Use herbal supports with each meal during this process, to
soothe the stomach and GI tract, and aid digestion: Ginger root,
licorice in small doses (500–2000 milligrams per day of undeglyc-

yrrhized root), slippery elm, and cardamom are herbs that can help. Nature's Answer makes a product called Bitters with Ginger drops suitable for children to aid digestion. Other products like this are available as well. Glycyrrhizin is the active component of licorice. It has antidepressant and anti-inflammatory effects, helps heal mucous membranes of the digestive tract, and may help heal ulcers. It can raise blood pressure in large doses, so only use very small doses. Children with a history of kidney problems may not be able to use this herb. Talk to a licensed pediatric naturopathic doctor (ND) if you have questions about how to use it. Licorice root solid extract is thick and gooey and black, and it tastes just like black licorice. Dissolve ⅛ to ¼ teaspoon licorice root extract in 4 to 6 ounces warm water and sip, to soothe the stomach. Reflux kids need to avoid IgG trigger foods while being weaned off their medication, to keep inflammation in the gut to a minimum. Following the prescription antifungal treatment, rotate *Saccharomyces boulardii* into the plan and give it at the opposite end of the day from your probiotic blend. Use this for a month, then switch to herbal antifungals. Eventually, your child should be able to get by on just the probiotic blend daily, and no reflux medication.

THE PICA KID

If you think your child eats a poor diet, you might be comforted to know that I've seen just about everything. This is my running list of strange stuff I have seen in food diaries. Kudos to those parents for telling me, because eating nonfood items, or "pica," is a classic sign of nutrition problems and disordered mineral status in particular. Many children with autism have pica. While some parents insist that the food diary look good so *they* look good, others threw that towel in long ago and just let it all hang out, which is more helpful for me as a clinician. Here are some examples of items children routinely swallowed. These were not fleeting oral tactile dalliances, but items that were regularly sought out with a vengeance by the child, with intent of full consumption: Paper clips. Sand. Dirty ice and snow, preferably licked from treads of shoes. Dirt. Pebbles. Feces, dog and human. Wooden toy trains, including the paint on them. Pencils. Erasers. Fabric. Plastic stuff. When I tell parents they can't surprise me on a food record, I mean it.

WHAT TO DO: First, have your pediatrician do routine screening for iron deficiency and lead toxicity. The iron screen should include not just hemoglobin and hematocrit, but transferrin, serum iron, and CBC also. This will be covered by insurance and give you fast, local guidance. If a child is urgently seeking nonfood items daily and eating them, there is a serious mineral imbalance that needs correcting. The child who licked trains in this vignette did turn out to have lead poisoning. He responded well to chelation therapy. Next, replenish minerals, especially zinc, selenium, molybdenum, magnesium, and chromium, to 100 percent daily value at least. Zinc in particular may need to be increased to 30 or more milligrams per day. Be cautious with copper supplementation if this is a child with autism. You might ask for a ceruloplasmin screen to be added on to the blood work for iron. If this child's diet is rigid for "yellow" food, milk, or opiate-forming foods, consider the GFCF diet, with the usual corrections up front for bowel flora. Yellow and milk diets are notoriously poor in minerals. Transitioning off this diet will be more healthful for your child in the long run.

THE BAD SLEEPER KID

There are bad sleepers at every age—babies, toddlers, and school-aged kids (not to mention adults). There are kids who at eleven years old are still cosleeping or needing a parent at their side every night in order to fall asleep. Cosleeping has its merits, but any parent needs breaks now and then. Your child should be able to grant you those. If this triggers meltdowns, it's time to intervene with some new strategies. Falling and staying asleep are blessed, precious, and necessary skills for people of all ages. Some nutrition problems can get in the way of this. Try fixing those before you torture your child with "Ferberization," which won't work when nutrition, neurotransmitter, or sensory modulation problems are in the way.

WHAT TO DO: For babies who can't fall asleep or stay asleep, first and foremost, give the most tolerable food source. If you have a reflux baby who isn't settling on breast milk and no one has slept in your house in six months, give up already! Check with your pediatrician, and switch to a hydrolysate formula option such as Nutramigen or Alimentum. These are stinky, I agree. But if your child needs a partially digested casein molecule in order to settle and progress, so be it. Add beneficial infant strains of Bifido and Lactobacillus to the feedings. If neither of these work, or your baby just hates them, try an elemental formula such as Neocate. Continue the probiotic. If that's no good, try the goat milk infant formula in Chapter 6. Soy formula may work, it may not; it is a toughie for most infants to digest. Breast milk is best for so many reasons, but if your baby is growing poorly and miserable, you are miserable, and everyone is mad and tired, it's not best anymore. Use a quarter cup Epsom salts nightly in the bath for sulfur and magnesium. Sulfur in particular is required to build nonpermeable junctions between villi in the intestine. This will help the baby's gut heal more quickly and tolerate feedings better, faster.

For toddlers and older kids, withdraw opiate-forming foods (gluten, casein, and possibly soy). These disrupt sleep cycles and may make kids wakeful in the middle of the night, causing them to be silly, tearful, or scared, and needing a parent's intervention. Make sure total calories are adequate. When they are low, this can also cause night wakings and crying. Young toddlers often revisit night crying because they are growing so fast that parents have not gotten up to speed on giving enough solid foods in the daytime. Use Epsom salts in nightly tubs, with lavender drops. Try herbal preparations for kids for better sleep, which usually include chamomile, passion flower, oatseed, nettles, or skullcap; avoid valerian and kava kava, as these may be habit-forming. Melatonin supplementation has helped many children with autism, who often seem to lack it. This is a hormone that regulates sleep. Use a sublingual spray such as ReadiSorb, starting with a 1-milligram dose and not exceeding 3 milligrams nightly. More melatonin can be safe and effective, but get guidance from your provider first. Make sure calcium is adequately supplemented, too. I usually recommend parents use an easy-to-absorb product such as Ionic Fizz calcium and magnesium before bed to aid sleep.

Some kids with sensory integration disorder still can't self-calm enough to fall asleep without help, even when all these nutrition supports are nicely in place. The nutrition parts can be adjunctive to sensory integration tricks, and the two can work together. If you have a Jacuzzi tub, older kids might benefit from the jets pounding on their skin before bed; younger ones can get in with you if this is not a major inconvenience. Other tricks are using a weighted blanket on the bed (quilted with plastic pellets inside), skin brushing and joint compressions at bedtime, or creating a bed that is like a small fort for your child, with lots of stuffed animals inside. White noise machines, fans, or even special music made to induce brain waves conducive to sleep can help. While this might seem like too much fuss and your child should just learn to sleep, if he just doesn't, consider the toll it is taking on you. If these things help your child sleep, and that helps you sleep, fine. It probably won't be necessary forever to use all these supports, and if it is, so what? Sleeping is better than not sleeping.

THE WORST-CASE SCENARIO KID

Is your child on a gastrotomy tube, developmentally delayed, not growing? This is a dire, sad, solitary, and traumatizing place to be as a parent and as a child. You have probably gotten some support from a major medical center for this unwanted journey. But if your child is still struggling, you need to make sure there is not a missing piece, not a stone left unturned. Some parents of children with autism, cystic fibrosis, or global developmental delay have walked out of this burning building of a parenting experience alive, with their children recovering and off the G-tube.

WHAT TO DO: First, if your child is on a G-tube and not progressing for growth, or if a G-tube has been left in for more than a year with no monitoring, call the doctor who put the tube in. Young toddlers with G-tubes should have a care plan with regular monitoring and a goal to wean them off the tube, or at least increase oral feeding. Next, make sure that what is going in the G-tube is food your child can tolerate. Rule this out with an ELISA panel that includes both IgE and IgG responses. If you are feeding an inflammatory food day in and day out, this can impede progress in a big way. Change to whatever formula or foods work better, and have your medical center's dietitian calculate for you the appropriate calories, proteins, fats, carbohydrates, and flow rate, using these new foods. If you get flack, give it. Sorry, but if these providers have left you hanging with no monitoring and no plan for improvement or weaning, you have every right to suggest a new plan and it is reasonable to have it considered by your team. Otherwise, perhaps they can suggest a different one? If your child is too young for reliable allergy testing and there are signs of intolerance (reflux, vomiting, shiners, frequent illness, irritable stools, eczema), then work backward from the major protein source. It is probably triggering inflammation; replace it.

Next, get a stool culture and check the bowel flora situation. Use a lab such as Doctor's Data that does full sensitivity testing and culture of both beneficial and detrimental species, not just a single smear for Clostridia or yeast. You may need to follow suggestions earlier in this chapter for reflux to correct this. If mucus is visible in vomit or stool, consider enzymes to break this up, such as Peptizyde, Fribrozym, or a prescription option. This will help the intestine absorb food better. The bottom line is that the entire digestive process may be compromised in a child on a gastrotomy tube, just as it is for a reflux kid. Forcing food in via a tube may not fix the problem at all, without correcting underlying obstacles to digestion and absorption. You should be absolutely sure a child with cystic fibrosis is not relying on inflammatory proteins day in and day out. Consider amino acid–based formulas or adding essential amino acids to the tube daily. Notable fats for easy absorption are ripe avocado and coconut milk. Use them as liberally as is tolerated to increase weight gain. You can also purchase medium-chain triglycerides (MCT oil), which are easy to digest and absorb, as a supplement and add these to the tube. Your hospital's dietitian or gastroenterologist may have a recommendation on MCT oil for you. It is available as an over-the-counter supplement and is safe to use (up to a tablespoon or so per day) unless your child has ketoacidosis or severe liver or lipid disorders, which always warrant close monitoring with a medical professional. Use carbohydrate sources allowable on SCD. These are the gentlest and easiest to absorb, and won't exacerbate yeast, Clostridia, or other disruptive microbes in the gut.

THE GROWTH HORMONE KID

These are children who have slipped off the growth chart, or are about to, and growth hormone injections have been suggested or are already being used. Though a full nutrition assessment is warranted, it usually has not been done.

WHAT TO DO: Request a nutrition consult, so growth and calorie intakes can be professionally assessed. As part of this assessment, ask for antigliadin IgG antibody testing as well as ELISA IgG for other foods. If it has not been done already, include ELISA IgE as well. If your child has an elevated IgG to several foods, and an elevated antibody titer for gliadin in particular, this may play a role in the growth failure or regression. If it is gluten sensitivity that is interfering with your child's growth, no matter how much growth hormone you inject, it won't fix the problem. That's not to say you will see no benefit from growth hormone, but it will not eradicate what might be the cause of the problem. Children vary. I have seen an in-range but high value for antigliadin IgG arrest growth in a two-year-old, and a highly above-range antigliadin IgG make apparently no impact on growth velocity in a very tall ten-year-old. The two-year-old immediately began growing on a gluten-free diet; the ten-year-old improved for focus and performance on a gluten-free diet. You will know if this matters in your child's case only if you do the test, then withdraw gluten completely, for at least four months.

Sounds obvious, but an adequate diet must be used during gluten withdrawal to yield diagnostically clear information. Don't put your child on a withering diet that is gluten-free, and expect it to permit growth. In my experience, children with positive gliadin antibody and growth regression/failure tend to have poor total calorie intakes—they simply don't eat enough, but that is not the sole cause for their lackluster growth. The error I see repeated by many a well-meaning GI doctor is assuming that gluten withdrawal will give the child less to eat, thus reducing food intake, when in fact, withdrawing gluten usually calms inflammation that interferes with appetite and absorption in these cases. When the gluten-free trial is done correctly, inflammation diminishes, reflux abates, appetite improves, and weight gain ensues—as long as the calorie intake is up to the correct level along with the gluten avoidance. The barrier for these children is that calorie intakes remain impossibly low as long as gluten is interfering and triggering inflammation, reflux, stomachaches, or other problems. As always, clearing the runway first with good bowel flora balance will speed things up.

With regard to all these strategies, adjust your developmental expectations timeline for your child. A child on the autism spectrum may take more time to work out potty training, even if bowel movements are more typical. A child with sensory integration disorder will use infantile helps longer, like pacifiers or bottles, for neurological organizing and self-soothing. A child with gross motor delays may need to begin solids a bit later or on a more gradual schedule, because babies need to sit up well and hold their heads up before they can safely begin chewing. School-aged children with special needs are no different. Finding the right balance of accommodation and challenge is unique to each child. Make sure that nutrition problems are not getting in the way, and use strategies that are scaffolded for success.

What to Expect from the Nutrition Care Process

Nutrition care is only as effective as its weakest piece. Unlike other interventions, it has many pieces that must be fit together gradually. Complete each step of the nutrition care process described earlier before adding the next one, or jumping in with another therapeutic modality. If one piece is left undone, it will slow or arrest progress. I give parents written care plans with explicit steps to follow, unique to their child; when the steps are followed in a timely way, there is more success. A common pitfall is expecting overnight changes or a pace for resolution akin to taking ibuprofen for a headache. Nutrition care can be a long haul; the goal is to replenish cells and tissues in your child that have been wanting, for years in some cases, for the right balance of nutrients. While early positive signs are common when starting a special diet, the whole situation doesn't get fixed in a week or two. It requires patience and commitment. While I have seen nonverbal, classically autistic children become verbal, conversational, and newly able in a classroom in a time span of a few months, this is usually the result of hard work and commitment to the nutrition piece by the family. These children have parents who, for whatever reason, are able to muster the energy to be very determined and focused, no small task when a child has special needs. These parents usually create good networks around themselves: family, grandparents, neighbors, support groups, child care providers so Mom and Dad can get a break, and health care providers who applaud their determination and devotion rather than undermine it by telling parents it is of no value. They are positive, positive, positive about their goals, their determination, and their outlook, and they seek to surround themselves with more of the same.

One other point that enhances success: While nutrition care works beautifully with other interventions, it is best to introduce only one new modality at a time. If other therapies (ABA, sensory integration, speech therapy, etc.) are in place already, then it is fine to add a new variable such as nutrition care. But it becomes confusing to introduce more than one new therapy at a time. Some parents like to dive in with every possible treatment as soon as the child is diagnosed with an autism spectrum disorder. They hold back nothing and begin speech therapy, sensory integration therapy, hippotherapy, social skills training, and a special diet all at once. While this is laudable, most parents find it exhausting after a month or two (imagine how the child feels!) and tend to drop some tools that may be extremely valuable in the big picture. Pace yourself, knowing that this is going to be a lifelong journey. Recovery does happen, but it is rare that a child is entirely free from needing any education supports or continued measures by the time he is eight or nine years old, if he starts out as a deeply affected toddler.

Getting Started and Getting Sick

One homeopathic tenet holds that getting sick at the start of treatment is a very good sign, so good that it has a name: the healing crisis. This is when the body completes its purge of a virus, trauma, illness, or even an emotional state that was supposedly arrested at some point. The intent of a homeopathic remedy, if the right one is chosen, is to reengage that purging momentum and process, and muster the body's own usual skills and tools to eradicate a disease condition, infectious agent, or illness. Another homeopathic tenet states that healing starts from the head and works its way down.

I've observed both these tenets in action with nutrition care, too. Nutrition therapies can trigger large physiological adjustments, including a bout of illness or irritability at first. Toxins that have been managed for months or years can begin to leave cells or fatty tissues in a hurry, out every possible exit, including urine, stool, skin, or breath. You may notice your child's breath, skin, hair, or eliminations smelling funny initially and transiently. Skin rashes are not uncommon, especially when viral or fungal material is finally being shed from the body, as it should be. A sudden ringworm rash can mean that yeast is on its way out, as long as the rash is transient, harmless (not hives or growing welts), and not sticking around beyond a couple days. This looks like round, reddish, coin-size circles with pale or white centers. Viral-looking rashes can pop out, too. They should come and go quickly, within a day or two or three. If these don't persist or cause serious discomfort, let them pass.

If you notice signs and symptoms moving downward on your child, from head to toe, encourage the process when reasonable, by not giving over-the-counter symptomatic treatments that suppress the body's efforts to purge toxins (pain and fever reducers, cold medicines, antihistamines) unless your child is uncomfortable or in danger. If you note rising hives, welts, hot fever, vomiting, or watery diarrhea, call your doctor. While children in my own caseload have sometimes shown dramatic expulsions like these in working their way out of an overload of viral, bacterial, fungal, or other toxins, keeping your doctor in the loop will help discern when to treat these and when to leave them be to work themselves out.

In my experience, nutrition supports shorten illness duration or help prevent illness altogether. During illness, children can use zinc up to 30 or 40 milligrams per day, vitamin C to bowel tolerance

(Emergen-C packets work well for kids), or vitamins A and D in cod liver oil, one tablespoon daily for up to a week. Herbal tools abound, for which you can consult a naturopathic doctor. Homeopathic remedies can help, too. If you don't have a homeopath but would like to explore this tool, add a copy of *Everybody's Guide to Homeopathic Medicines* to your home library. This is an excellent book that helps parents safely and effectively treat minor fevers, illnesses, bumps, and scrapes from early infancy. If your child is really uncomfortable or you are really concerned, call your doctor.

It is not unusual for a child to revisit an illness once the diet removes inflammatory foods. It's as though the immune system is finally unburdened enough to direct its energy toward a harbored agent—a respiratory virus, a bacterial infection in the ear—what have you. When parents call to say the child is sick soon after we begin, I take this as a positive sign. It is usually the last illness the child has for a long while after repeat illnesses and infections have been a problem, and it signals a regrouping of resources in the immune system. If this happens to your child and an antibiotic is needed, see if a concomitant prescription for Nystatin can be allowed, or a follow-up prescription for a drug such as fluconazole. These will quickly target yeast that the antibiotic encourages to excess. Follow these with probiotic supports to replenish health bowel bacteria. If no antifungal treatment is permitted, be sure you move in quickly with high-potency probiotics.

It can be overwhelming for parents to discern what is causing what when several therapies are begun at once. Big transitions (new school, tutoring program, different sitter, illness in Mom or Dad) and new therapies for speech, motor, or behavior that demand more of your child may trigger oppositional behavior at first, too. If your child is using some therapies already, therapists in these other modalities can become good observers of progress from nutrition measures. They typically begin reporting leaps and bounds for language, motor skills, or behavior, once the nutrition piece is added, which helps you refine and prioritize your child's total care plan. The more support you can garner from your child's provider team, including your pediatrician, biomedical provider, or primary MD provider, the easier it will be to stick with it. If you are confused about how to proceed with your child's special diet intervention, revisit the sequence suggested in Chapter 2.

There will be times when your efforts with the diet just don't seem to be paying off. Perhaps your child doesn't eat enough, or eats too much of the wrong stuff. This is where it may help to use medical nutritionals, discussed in the next chapter, along with supplements. Don't forget that you are using a relatively unwieldy medical intervention and doing your best. Revisit your support and provider networks as often as you need to for more guidance.

FIVE

Supplements

Medical Foods and Making Sense of a Dizzying Array of Options

Functional Nutrients, Nutraceuticals, and Medical Foods: What Are Those?

You're not alone if you are feeling dazed by the thousands of supplement choices tossed around for children with developmental, learning, or behavioral diagnoses. Used judiciously, supplements can help children improve on many levels. As with most facets of nutrition care, you are probably not hearing much about this from your pediatrician. How to supplement a child with special needs is a ballooning field in itself. Inexplicably, to my knowledge, there is no accredited specialization offered in this for licensed nutrition professionals, naturopathic doctors, or physicians, which is astounding, given the enormity of the supplement industry. The pharmaceutical industry, which is a larger behemoth in comparison, is present at every step of the physician's training, funding clinical trials, providing free products, writing fact sheets, underwriting training activities. Doctors get thoroughly trained in the prescribing of medications, but there is little professional continuity for how to use supplements.

During my studies in the 1970s and 1980s, supplementation was considered foolish by mainstream medicine. One of my undergraduate professors repeatedly joked that all it did was make expensive urine. It was presumed that food alone could and should adequately meet nutritional needs for most adults, and certainly for all infants and children. We were all actually supposed to eat that well. Orthomolecular medicine was rising then; it touted megadose supplementation as medicine, but did not gain a deep toehold in the mainstream landscape. Even naturopathic doctors, who train in the medicinal use of natural substances such as supplements and herbs, do not have a specialization or certification for pediatric special needs. You can go to any type of MD specialist under the sun, and registered dietitians and nurses can get certification in various pediatric disciplines. But how do you find the right resource for supplementing your special-needs child? Do our children need this?

I now respectfully disagree with the nutritional biochemistry professor who joked about making expensive urine. Nutrition science and practice have come a long way since 1980 (maybe that professor has, too). Recommendations for daily intakes of each nutrient are created with population and clinical data that is crunched by panels of experts at the Food and Nutrition Board of the Institute of Medicine. The data used is derived mostly from infants and children who are healthy, and the recommendations yielded by the data are intended to maintain health under normal circumstances, not treat specific conditions. Yes, the children I have encountered with special needs usually do need supplements, at least initially. Malabsorption, inflammation, toxicity, and marginal dietary intakes are not normal. A normal diet cannot overcome these problems, which can disrupt cellular chemistry, growth, and whole body physiology. Medications do not always do this job very well; they often appear to do a lesser job than the natural substances can do, since they are only masking symptoms and do not usually correct an underlying problem. Sometimes a combination of meds and supplements is the trick. While this is a fast-emerging area of practice, it is evident that supplementation can help overcome and redirect problems that the "one in six" kids have. This is what functional nutrients do, and a role like this for a nutrient was not widely recognized around 1980, when my professor joked about the futility of supplements. He was thinking of typical healthy individuals with no disease process when he said that. And he couldn't foresee all the nutritional biochemistry work to come in years ahead, which would begin to tease apart the behavior of nutrients in chronic conditions such as cancer, anxiety, depression, inflammatory bowel disease, and autoimmune disorders.

Essential nutrients are those we know to be absolutely necessary in diets, for human life. Functional foods and nutrients are those that can confer a health benefit, such as disease prevention, tissue building, or enhanced mood, cognition, or physical performance. An essential nutrient may take on a new, functional role at high doses in certain disease conditions. While children with entrenched struggles such as autism appear to need replenishment for basic nutrition more often than we previously knew, many have enjoyed benefits from therapeutically dosed supplements that medications could never have conferred. Since these are often natural substances, they are not patentable, and thus don't draw consistent interest for clinical trials. No one can make as much money selling supplements as they can by patenting and selling pharmaceuticals. Scientific review of supplements is scant compared to pharmaceuticals—not because this is an invalid area of clinical review, but because there is no way to own exclusive rights to the findings. The dominance of pharmaceuticals in our medical culture may be experiencing a shift, as consumers have more success with natural substances, and more interest and demand for them. Combination products—medications with supplements in one—are probably not far off. Nutraceuticals, or nutrients dosed for pharmacologic effect, are growing in popularity, too. Not to mention medical foods.

What's a medical food? This is a product specially formulated to replace food as a major treatment for a specific condition. It is intended to confer a therapeutic benefit, such as repairing gut tissue and reducing inflammation in the bowel. Technically, medical foods are to be used with professional supervision, and their labels must state that they are intended to manage a specific disorder or condition. They are supposed to meet the nutritional requirements of said condition, based on existing science. Examples of medical foods are Ultra-Inflam-X and Ultracare for Kids (both made by Metagenics), which provide calories, protein, fats, and carbs, along with some vitamins, minerals, and functional nutrients or herbs. These are powders that you mix in the fluid of your choice; they are "food" because you can use them as a meal replacement or adjunct to a meal.

The Story of EO28/Splash

I began using medical foods in 1999, when I first encountered a product from the United Kingdom called Neocate. This medical food is a ready-to-drink, amino acid–based formula for children with multiple food intolerances and/or inflammatory bowel disease. It provides all essential amino acids in a ready-to-absorb form. Because the protein source in Neocate is not made from a naturally occurring, intact protein molecule, but from individual amino acids, there is nothing in the protein source that can trigger more inflammation. This was what my own child, then nearly three, needed at the time. I began using this product for him as an adjunct to his restricted diet. It worked very well. His growth quickly improved. He relied on this product into second grade. I began suggesting it in my practice, where it worked well for other children, too. It seemed to enhance developmental progress for children with autism who were using special diets.

The company that makes this product makes several specialized medical foods for infants and children. This one was a favorite since it came in a ready-to-drink, juice box format. Neocate underwent a name change and soon became EO28. Years ago, when my practice was in Massachusetts, I would twist the arm of the regional sales representative for samples of EO28, which was normally seen only on pediatric gastroenterology wards—not in a pediatrician's office and certainly not in an office like mine. Most pediatricians had never heard of it, which I discovered when trying to enlist their support in authorizing its use. It does not require a prescription, but because it is expensive and is not needed except in situations where other foods are intolerable, a physician's prescription can help get it covered by insurance in some cases. I gave samples to families who might most benefit, and did the paperwork pro bono so it could be covered by insurance for these children— as it should have been. These children were not able to use soy, casein, gluten, or hydrolysate formulas. Some had an allergy or sensitivity to egg, beef, fish, and so on, or they usually refused meats due to texture objections. Most of them were nutritionally struggling because they could not eat enough protein, or normally absorb the protein they did eat. Some of them could use another product called Pepdite, which is a hydrolysate (partly broken down) soy protein formula that incorporates hyrdolysate protein from pork also. Sounds horrible, but some children took well to it and were better off for it. For the children for whom I recommended EO28 or Pepdite, it was usually the only safe and reliably eaten source of high-quality protein they could use. Without an option like EO28, they were at risk for remaining in nutritional failure, or tumbling into it. "Nutritional failure" is a clinically explicit term with clear criteria, based on growth patterns. I had often seen nutritional failure in children with autism in my practice. Not only did EO28 turn this around for children using special diets, it appeared to boost the developmental benefit of a special diet protocol. It is a very appropriate application for a medical food.

I quietly continued providing EO28 to families who would try it for years. I was always grateful to Susie Gingrich, RD, the dietitian who generously left me samples knowing that I wasn't going to be placing a large order, or any order. I was simply getting this stuff out to families who had no other options. If it got covered by insurance, great—at least I knew the child would have a means to be fed adequately while we worked other measures for gut healing. I spent a lot of time writing letters of request for insurance coverage and convincing pediatricians that this would be the best option.

In the summer of 2007, a marketing firm called me and asked if a representative could meet me. It was a representative for Nutricia North America, the company that makes EO28. EO28 was now called "Splash," and they had heard that it was helpful for children with autism—which was basically an off-label use of it. "Off-label" is the practice of using a prescription drug outside the scope of its FDA-approved label—such as when Singulair, approved for asthma, was found to also be effective for GI inflammation. EO28 was a medical food approved for certain GI conditions, not autism. They wanted to know what I was doing with EO28, how many children with autism had used it under my guidance, and what happened. Eventually they had me review my case files for kids with autism who had used their products. It turned out that I had attempted EO28 or Pepdite with one hundred children. Apparently I was just about the only person they could dig up, or one of very few, who had thorough records on this sort of thing.

I knew this formula had helped a lot, but reviewing my case studies surprised even me. Many families liked this stuff, but couldn't keep using it without insurance coverage due to its high cost. Other kids just never liked it. But I was able to track down a few families I had not spoken to in years who'd been able to stay with it. Without question, children who had used a restricted diet for autism with EO28 did better, developmentally and for growth parameters, than children who used a restricted diet without it. At least one of the children was described as fully recovered by his mom. Her son was a typically complex and difficult case when I met him at age two. He had growth regression; an autism diagnosis; neurological quirks such as toe walking, nystagmus, and walking in circles; excessively mobile joints; gross motor delays; extreme anxiety; sensory integration disorder; and chronically irritable bowel mixed with constipated stools. He ended up using EO28 for about five years as an adjunct to his restricted diet. When I worked with him, from ages two to four, it had afforded a swift recovery of a normal growth pattern and increased his developmental tasking. It was clearly a big help. I knew the nutrition care piece was going well, but this was not a kid I ever expected would do a horizon job on an autism diagnosis. He now attends a regular classroom, rides a bike, is learning to ski, is reciprocally social, and has friends.

That's quite a claim. A clinical trial is under way to test Splash's efficacy in autism. Even if I had never met anyone at Nutricia, I would still feel compelled to mention this medical food, for two reasons: One, in spite of some objectionable ingredients, on balance, it is a serviceable tool whose benefits usually outweigh its drawbacks. As so often happens in the pharmaceutical world, a product developed for one purpose ends up being great for another. This is true for Splash. The product needs improvement to be fully dependable and successful for children with autism, but it's on the right track. Two, so far, nobody else makes a competing product in this ready-to-feed format. There are free amino acid powders available for kids that mix with water or juice. But these are more like supplements than medical foods, because they don't provide complete nutrition, and don't address the calorie malnutrition so common in children using special diets for autism. Nutricia also nailed the format—a juice box. It's ready to drink. Your kid can bring it to school in his lunch, or anywhere else. It doesn't have to be mixed or refrigerated ahead of time. Despite its packaging, it is not juice. It has the protein equivalent of milk, in a safe, free amino acid form; more calories per ounce than milk; all essential vitamins and minerals; and easy-to-absorb forms of fats and carbohydrate. For kids with multiple food intolerances, inflammatory bowel diseases, nutritional failure, or cystic fibrosis, it can be a great tool.

The Importance of Classroom Calories

Children need calories throughout the day. School performance is linked to calorie, protein, and micronutrient intakes in children. Yet many schools are now so squeezed to accommodate curriculum requirements that lunch periods have shrunk to as few as ten minutes to actually sit down and eat. This is a lot to ask of a very efficient and focused child, let alone one with attention issues or other special needs. Parents often tell me, as we are reviewing food diaries, that their children with special needs do not eat at school. For children with sensory processing issues, lunch can be a nightmare. Too loud, too fast, too crazy; the environment is overwhelming and many children freeze up or become hyperactive to compensate for being overwhelmed. They often simply do not eat in this commotion. Their performance by afternoon can be abysmal; they can't focus or pay attention, or they dissolve into tears or tantrums. This can be entirely due to a calorie deficit in the context of the special-needs diagnosis. A typical child may become disengaged or less focused in this situation, but a child with special needs may simply shut down, fall asleep, or melt down. Some will hold it together until they are home, and then explosive behaviors ensue; many parents have seen that the only remedy is food. If this is your child, a portable, nutritious tool like Splash may be a good way to divert this. Splash is also an easy bargaining chip for parents and school staff: Finish this drink, and you can have XYZ. For children in calorie malnutrition, this can quickly overcome energy deficits that slow or impair learning, developmental tasking, sleep, wound healing, mitochondrial function, or gut tissue healing.

A product like this is also a convenient way to avoid calorie malnutrition for kids who fail with other foods, and an effective way to replenish protein when other foods trigger inflammation. But another important benefit for children with autism who use Splash is that it has been shown, in studies on children with Crohn's disease, to reverse intestinal permeability. Restoring normal gut function is a foundation piece for the child with autism. Once the intestine can resume some normal functioning, all the nutrients needed for growth, learning, and development can get to where they are supposed to go—and children function better, learn better, socialize better, grow better. Besides its potential for reversing intestinal permeability, Splash is ready to absorb. It requires nothing of the human gut in terms of digestion, which we already know is challenging for children with autism. The nutrients in it are ready to take across the intestinal wall and go to work. The amino acids your child needs to build neurotransmitters are there, ready for service. There is no inflammatory response triggered; there are no polypeptides malabsorbed and no dietary opiates locking on to endorphin receptors in the brain. The amino acids in Splash can also go to work in gut tissue repair, another job that needs high-value protein efficiently loosed from foods in order to get done. With Splash, the building blocks of protein are at the ready. Your child does not have to digest them first. Children with autism using Splash still need individualized supplement protocols, but this is a big improvement over rice milk, which is nutritionally vacant, or Peptamen Junior, which uses casein hydrolysate as a protein source.

More research will tell the story. Watching how a child's demeanor and ability change when he is fully nourished, and when the veil of dietary opiates is lifted, is always an eye-opener. It's easy to assume that a child's lassitude, lethargy, disengaged demeanor, tantrums, rigidity, and blank countenance are entirely due to his autism—until you see all of these shift with good nutrition interventions. Splash, Pepdite, and Neocate One Plus are the only products available so far that are nutritionally complete medical foods in a ready-to-feed, easy-to-absorb format.

Is Splash Right for Your Child?

If this stuff is so great, why isn't everyone using it? It has been around for years, and so have special diets for autism that exclude gluten, casein, or soy. Parents are always looking for an easy way to give their children a nutritious dairy alternative, and Splash is just that. So why can't we just go buy it in the baby formula aisle? Besides being a United Kingdom–based company that does not have much name recognition in the United States, Nutricia is new to direct consumer marketing. Their products have historically been placed in the hands of physicians in hospitals, or medical scientists doing clinical trials, not moms and dads surfing the Net. But a bigger problem, as of this writing, is that Splash, Neocate One Plus, and Pepdite have some ingredients that are poorly tolerated in some cases. For some children with autism, these ingredients are too challenging, making Splash an option they probably can't use. This may change in the future, but so far, many parents and providers object to some of the artificial ingredients in it. Now that I've enumerated the benefits, here are some of the challenges that children with autism may face when trying Splash:

It contains L-aspartate. This is a naturally occurring, nonessential amino acid, also called aspartic acid. It is an excitatory neurotransmitter, like glutamate. It can overstimulate receptors for N-methyl D-aspartate (NMDA) in the brain, causing a flood of calcium ions into nerve cells, which is highly damaging to cell structures. NMDA receptors allow electrical signals to pass between neurons. When they are activated, they are open, permitting calcium ions and electrical signals to pass unmitigated. This can play a role in seizures. I know of no records of Splash triggering seizures, but foods with excitotoxins such as NutraSweet (which is metabolized to aspartate) and MSG (monosodium glutamate) have been linked to seizure events in some cases. Children with autism—about a third of whom also have seizure disorders—have been noted to have too much glutamate in their brain tissue to begin with, so heavy reliance on a medical food that may exacerbate this is problematic. Out of over one hundred children with autism who have tried Splash under my care, two have reported marked behavioral agitation, disintegration, or rageful behavior within an hour or two of drinking it. These children may have been extremely sensitive to the free aspartate in Splash. In children who need three or four boxes daily (up to 32 ounces), this may be problematic and cumulative. Neocate One Plus also contains both aspartate and glutamine, which can play a role in overstimulating NMDA receptors, or in shifting the ratio of glutamate to GABA away from the more calming GABA.

One natural compound with promise for negating this effect is a supplement called N-acetyl-cysteine, or NAC. NAC is a precursor to glutathione in the body, a compound we rely on for detoxification and for heavy metals clearing (we already know that glutathione is imbalanced in conditions such as autism and schizophrenia). NAC is a standard emergency room treatment for Tylenol overdose in infants and children. It is very safe and effective for that application. NAC is currently in review with at least three clinical trials as of this writing, for its use in mitigating obsessive-compulsive disorders or autism features. It has already shown clinical effectiveness for some features of schizophrenia. The mechanism of action for this may relate to regulation of NMDA receptors and glutathione chemistry. Children in the studies have been given NAC up to a dose of 40 milligrams per kilogram per day and safety at high doses is so far looking good. But because NAC can make stored heavy metals migrate, it can be tricky to use without oversight from a clinician knowledgeable about chelation. Check with a provider experienced in this before using NAC on a daily basis in doses above 500 milligrams per day.

If your child becomes agitated, upset, or hyperactive on Splash, you may be seeing effects of excitotoxins. You may be able to interrupt this by giving your child NAC (200–500 milligrams), or carnosine (200 milligrams), two amino acids that show promise for mitigating activity at

NMDA receptors. If you find that either reverses a picture of excitotoxicity after Splash, share this with your doctor or biomedical provider. It is possibly confirming glutamate neurotoxicity or NMDA receptor malfunction, which may point to a new treatment path for your child. Psychological features of ongoing NMDA receptor malfunction can include anxiety, obsessive-compulsive disorders, paranoia, repetitive behaviors, and cognitive rigidity.

Other than aspartate, some of the challenging ingredients in Splash are the ones that help make it so effective: maltodextrin and free amino acids. Some disruptive bowel bacteria can usurp free amino acids just as others take carbohydrates. Splash uses corn-sourced maltodextrin as a carbohydrate source. This is gluten-free and easy to absorb, requiring minimal digestion. Maltodextrin is not allowed on the Specific Carbohydrate Diet (SCD), so anyone working strictly within SCD parameters won't want to use Splash. Most kids with autism tolerate this well, *if*, and this is a big if, they have bowel flora balanced first. If not, the carbohydrate source in Splash is eagerly lapped up by Candida and disruptive bowel flora. Maltodextrin from corn would not normally be a very big concern, since it usually pops up in processed foods in small amounts. But because children may use a lot of Splash daily, it means they may get a lot of maltodextrin. Splash also has sugar as a carbohydrate source, and Neocate One Plus relies on corn syrup solids. While gluten-free, all of these can cause disruptive flora to grow to excess and excrete toxic organic acids, which in turn can reach the brain, impairing behavior, sleep, or cognition, or triggering agitation.

Children who use these products successfully do better when probiotic supplementation and antifungal rotations are in place, but then so do most children with autism. Ideally, use aggressive bowel flora corrections before using Splash on a daily basis. If your child tries Splash and quickly becomes hyper, silly, unfocused, or disruptive, it may be due to untreated bowel flora that just got a boost.

Lastly, Splash, Neocate One Plus, and Pepdite have artificial flavors that can be objectionable for children who have difficulty with phenolic compounds. You may see red tips of ears or cheeks in your child if this is the case, and the Epsom salts in the bath are usually an effective fix. These formulas also rely on omega-6 oils as part of their fat source. They overlook omega-3 fats, which are now so well known for their benefits that they are common in everything from other medical foods, to supplements, eggs, breakfast cereals, infant formula, and even some brands of orange juice.

If You Want to Try Splash

Because children with autism may need a medical food in large amounts daily, it would be preferable if all these ingredients were optimized. This is a big food science challenge, since ideal ingredients can just plain taste bad, spoil too fast, or refuse to mix together, resulting in an expensive product that nobody likes. In any case, some view the ingredient objections I've mentioned here as hairsplitting, and maintain that the very large needs of children in nutritional failure supersede these problems. My experience with Splash has satisfied me that, for the most part, it is worth some trouble to see if a child can succeed with it. It can be an effective bridge piece between the early phase of a special diet, when few foods are accepted or tolerated and nutritional failure must be reversed, to the later phases, when children are eating better and can digest more foods, more typically. Its clinical benefits have been reviewed already and are undergoing further review. If it is well tolerated, it will replenish your child nutritionally, and may trigger some reversal of intestinal permeability. Parents can concoct their own versions of a nutritionally complete medical food with all natural ingredients, but this would be a Herculean task in bench chemistry that your child may simply throw on the floor. Smoothies with essential amino acids and some extra vitamins are reasonable to offer, but are still not nutritionally complete; suggestions for smoothies can be found in the next chapter.

If you want to try Splash, manage the challenges that come with it by first making sure bowel flora are in good standing; by having passed through opiate withdrawal before introducing it; and by using Epsom salts with baking soda in baths daily. Treating bowel flora first, as you should anyway when beginning a special diet for your child, will enhance absorption of Splash into your child rather than into middle-man gut bugs. Give a small amount (4–8 ounces) and watch for tolerance. Splash should not cause rashes or hives. In fact, it is fre-quently used for children to relieve dermatitis from foods. If you notice redness in your child's cheeks or ears, this may indicate a sulfa-tion deficit worsened by Splash. This can be quickly redirected with an Epsom salt bath, which permits swift uptake of magnesium sulfate. Sulfur is needed for many functions in digestion, for absorption, and for liver enzymes that detoxify chemicals, drugs, or toxins. Besides arti-ficial flavorings that some children may not manage well, if your child has bowel flora that Splash triggered, this may send an overwhelming load of organic acids from these flora to the liver for detoxification. This may overwhelm the liver's sulfation capacity. Epsom salts, a cup or two in a bath, can help. Children who are still noshing on dietary opiates (wheat, dairy, and soy foods every day) usually reject Splash outright, for the same reason they reject any other food: It doesn't cre-ate any opiates. For that reason, it is preferable to introduce Splash after you have completely removed dietary opiates and your child is no longer accustomed to having them.

Quite often, children new to Splash don't like it. If your child's diet is routinely inadequate for total calories and protein, it is worth working with Splash for a bit to see if you can win your child over. Rewards for trying something new can work well—give your child a favorite activity or item after she tries a few ounces. Children who are milk-addicted often reject Splash because it is formulated to resemble a fruit smoothie or juice, not a milk drink. These children might take better to Neocate or Pepdite powdered formulas, which have a milky consis-tency and appearance, but are nutritionally equivalent to Splash. None of these products works well when mixed with foods or fluids besides water. Follow package instructions and use them as directed. You may be able to transition a child off milk slowly, by reconstituting Neocate or Pepdite per package instructions, then mixing it with milk in gradually larger and larger amounts, until the entire drink is Neocate or Pepdite. Mixing these powders directly with milk or juice doesn't work well.

TRANSITIONING OFF MILK AND ONTO SPLASH

- Children with autism spectrum disorders usually do not like changes in routines. Changing what they eat is a big one. As is true with any big transition for your child, your demeanor and attitude are very important. Your child will sense this and will follow your lead. Children with autism may take longer than typical children to accept an unwanted transition, but they can do it. Keep a calm, neutral demeanor; present new foods, including Splash, with little fanfare.

- Young children do not need to know why Splash or any other new food is being offered, and they do not need to agree with your rationale for it. Older or higher-functioning children can be offered information as they ask for it; let their questions lead you.

- Too much detail about autism, food allergy, or bowel problems is unnecessary and may heighten a child's anxiety. Present this change as you would any other needed change and have confidence in your decision.

- This strategy works best as part of a total diet strategy. If your child still eats cheese, yogurt, ice cream, and other dairy foods, he may be more likely to refuse Splash.

- Expect some defiance and tantrums. Many children reject Splash at first, especially those who use milk as a main calorie and protein source or those still eating a lot of wheat and dairy foods.

- Many parents describe their children with autism as "addicted" to milk, cheese, and starchy wheat foods. There is some scientific evidence to back up that observation, so keep this in mind as you withdraw these favorites from your child, and be ready to be patient.

- Your child may actually experience withdrawal symptoms that are unpleasant. These pass more quickly when you adhere to the diet restriction; giving "a little" wheat or dairy food will provoke and prolong withdrawal symptoms.

- To enhance and hasten your child's acceptance of Splash, if possible, optimize your child's bowel flora before you begin. Talk to your provider about using antifungal therapy if your child has had antibiotics.

- Your child's first tries at Splash should be at home when there are few demands on both of you. This lets you observe how it is tolerated.

- If Splash makes your child have unwanted behavior changes, this may signal a need for antifungal therapy before using Splash, or it may signal poor tolerance of excitotoxins in Splash or Neocate products.

Other Medical Foods

There are many powdered products available for children, from free amino acids powders like AminoPlex, to mixtures such as Ultracare for Kids that include substantial calories, vitamins, and minerals. Some of these are medical foods, some are supplements. It becomes a medical food when it can replace actual food and when it is being used to treat a specific condition. Medical foods work best when used as recommended, for their recommended purpose, and as a transitional chapter in a child's special diet progression. Keep in mind the long-term goal of the medical food: to create enough gut tissue recovery and nutritional replenishment so that your child can start eating more real food and tolerate it well. Products such as Boost, Peptamen Junior, Nutramigen, Alimentum, or Carnation Instant Breakfast are not suitable for GFCF diets since the protein in all of these is based on either casein or casein hydrolysate. These are too close to the casein-sourced opiate peptides that children on the spectrum absorb to excess from the gut.

As for powdered medical foods such as Ultracare for Kids, or free amino acid powder supplements, children frequently object to the feel of a gritty powder in their foods or drinks. But if your child doesn't mind, these support good total nutrition while your child uses a special diet. Some manufacturers avoid artificial flavors and colors in their products, which can be easier to tolerate for many children. Start with a small amount in a new smoothie recipe and see how it goes. It may backfire to add a new item such as a medical food powder to something your child loves to eat every day—they will detect, and often reject, the change you've made. Rather than mess with their existing success, make a new item and test it out. Check labels for these products to make sure that you are not redundantly dosing micronutrients.

Starting, Adding, and Mixing Supplements

There are two tiers to supplementation: One is replenishment of baseline normal nutrition status, which products like Splash can do well. Both medical foods and broad-spectrum, high-potency mulitvitamin and mineral supplements are useful for this first tier. Nearly all "one in six" children I encounter need replenishment in this regard, before moving on to the second tier. The second tier is using specific supplements in therapeutic doses, as pharmacologic agents, or nutraceuticals. When and how to add those can be reliably planned using clinical signs and symptoms. Lab data is a helpful fill-in that is not always absolutely necessary to define an effective supplement plan. See "The Nutrition-Focused Physical Exam" in Chapter 3 to review which nutrients may be marginal for your child. Young children quickly show deficits for nutrients in skin, hair, behavior, sleep, growth patterns, tongue, teeth, lips, and nails. Sometimes the signs on the child suggest deficit status for a nutrient, while the lab value remains in a low-normal range. As always, treatment choices should be based on the whole child, not the lab data alone. This information usually gives enough to begin a baseline supplement protocol, without lab studies. After using baseline replenishments for a few weeks, revisit the signs and symptoms, and consider lab data to refine what may work best at a therapeutic dose.

If nothing else, start with a high-potency vitamin and mineral supplement such as Kirkman's Chewable Multivitamin and Mineral Wafer, or Klaire Labs VitaSpectrum (powder or capsules). There are now countless choices marketed to children with autism. Whatever you choose should be easy for your child to take (there are capsules, chewables, liquids, powders, sublingual and nasal sprays, and topicals), and it should provide full daily recommended values for your child's age for the entire B vitamin group and for zinc. It should also give at least half the daily value for selenium, chromium, manganese, iodine, molybdenum, and vitamins A, C, D, E, and K. The full daily value is useful for children with poor rigid diets, at least until they are able to reliably eat food sources of minerals. Some magnesium is helpful in a multi, too, though it is also supplemented effectively with calcium at bedtime, as this approach may help sleep. Avoid multis with a full daily value for copper if your child has autism, since copper excess is not unusual in these children. Some kids may also not do well with iron supplements, but if your child has dark circles under the eyes, pallor, redness at the belly button, and lassitude or is quick to fatigue, you should check his iron status with your pediatrician.

Some multis for "one in six" kids include megadoses of some of nutrients. A popular example is pyridoxine (vitamin B6) or pyridoxal-5-phosphate (P5P, a metabolically active form of B6). Unless lab work (usually a urine organic acid test) corroborates that this will matter, it is prudent to replenish it to a baseline level first, either at or perhaps double the daily recommended intake (DRI) value. Higher-dose B6 or P5P can be nicely supportive of brain chemistry for autism but can also make children agitated, hyper, and wakeful if they are given more than they need (and they do sometimes need very high doses to improve). The oft-heard advice is to start low, go slow, and give new items in the morning so no one loses a night's sleep in case there is a reaction. B vitamins are excreted quickly and are unlikely to become toxic. If they are given to problematic excess, this resolves with stopping the vitamin.

Certain forms of vitamins and minerals are more effective for circumstances such as toxicity, poor absorption, leaky gut, inflammation, and oxidative stress. P5P is an example; zinc picolinate is another (versus other forms of zinc). There are many applications for preferred forms of supplements, and your provider should help with which ones to use when. A few more examples of preferred forms are:

ORDINARY FORM	PREFERRED FORM	BECAUSE . . .
Oral cyanocobalamin (B12)	Methylcobalamin (B12), injected, inhaled, or sublingual	Repairs methylation deficits; overcomes poor intestinal absorption when administered other than orally.
Trans-palmitate (synthetic vitamin A)	Cis-palmitate (natural vitamin A)	Taken into rod cells of retina where it may engage frontal vision; no conversion from trans form is necessary.
Calcium carbonate	Elemental calcium, calcium citrate, calcium gluconate, or calcium glycinate	Calcium carbonate buffers stomach acid, which may already be too buffered in some children; it is also poorly absorbed.
Folic acid	Folate or folinic acid	Already methylated form; does not require methylation to function in cells.
Magnesium citrate, magnesium oxide	Magnesium taurinate, magnesium glycinate, or elemental magnesium	Less triggering of diarrhea.
Ferrous sulfate (iron)	Ferrous bis-glycinate	Less constipating, less irritating to stomach, better absorbed.

Getting a Better Multi

Most kids' multivitamins on supermarket and drugstore shelves—products such as Gummi Vits or ordinary children's chewables—do not use preferred forms of these nutrients, nor are they potent enough for the "one in six" kids, whose diets are notoriously poor for minerals and who must usually overcome malabsorption or deficits in cellular chemistry that convert vitamins and minerals to their bioactive forms. They also may not give adequate profiles of the B vitamin group, for which most of our kids have a heightened need. Children on gluten-free diets need good-quality B group support, too, since most wheat foods are fortified with B vitamins in the United State while foods made with other grains or tubers (rice, quinoa, tapioca, manioc, potato) are not. The many dysregulated facets of immune function, toxicity, and inflammation, plus poor diets, warrant broad-spectrum supplementation in most kids using a special diet. Most can progress well with a high-potency basic multi, and up to perhaps four or five other items each day to trigger therapeutic effects. More than this starts to get impractical, complicated, and difficult to comply with. While there may be periods, especially early on, when more items might be indicated, eventually your child should be recovering to the point where it becomes a manageable routine with just a few supplement items. A typical scenario might be giving your child a multi daily, plus two or three teaspoons of fish oils, a therapeutic item such as a methylcobalamin spray or shot three times a week, and perhaps additional zinc, calcium, and magnesium in a single powder. Or some children may do fine with that multi, Epsom salts and baking soda nightly in the bath, fish oils, and melatonin spray at bedtime for sleep. Each child is different, so allow yourself some time to introduce items that seem appropriate. If you are not seeing the progress you expect, engage your provider network for advice, guidance, and troubleshooting.

Therapeutic Dosing

How to give which supplements, in which forms, and at what doses can be refined with lab data in some cases, but quite often, you simply have to trial a supplement in a child to see if it is going to yield a benefit. The options are almost unlimited. I will repeat that no supplement can do its job completely if your child is in a chronic dietary deficit for calories, protein, or fats. If all signs indicate that a particular supplement ought to do something wonderful for your child and it just doesn't, go back to square one and make sure the total diet is adequate and the bowel flora are in balance. There are thousands of supplements literally at your fingertips on the Web. Instead of marching through them, I group them below by the issues that they are typically used to address in children on special diets. Items in the left column are those that can be safely tried at home, while those on the right show promise clinically but might be better monitored by a licensed health care professional with knowledge and experience in using supplements for children. Trying one item at a time is recommended, as opposed to using all at once.

Nutrition Supports for Seizure Control: Can Supplements Mitigate Seizures?

Seizures can be caused by head trauma, toxicity, low blood sugar, infection, low oxygen, or a metabolic imbalance. Children who use tools that correct toxicity burden, nutrition deficits, and metabolic abnormalities may see improvement in seizure control. Anecdotally, children in my own caseload have experienced this with aggressive corrections to disruptive bowel flora, like Candida, Clostridia, and others—thus supporting the possibility that toxins created by overgrowth of these microorganisms may overwhelm the brain in children with intestinal permeability. Others see improvement or resolution with high-dose pyridoxine (vitamin B6, which is needed to convert glutamate to GABA in the brain—see below), magnesium replenishment, and balancing of copper and zinc in the body. At least one child in my caseload stopped having "absence" seizures once dietary opiate sources (gluteomorphin and casomorphin) were no longer detectable in her urine.

Still other possibilities are emerging: Two promising natural modulators of excitotoxicity in the brain mentioned earlier are carnosine, an amino acid that can push GABA production, and N-acetyl cysteine, a precursor to glutathione. GABA (gamma-aminobutyric acid) is a calming chemical that has an inhibitory influence on nerve cells; its activity at nerve cell receptor sites may be involved for a child with anxiety disorders or epilepsy. As was also noted earlier in this chapter, children with autism appear to have too much glutamate in their brain tissue. Excitotoxic levels of glutamate are normally balanced by conversion to calming GABA, a biochemical step that requires vitamin B6. This is one reason why many children with autism may benefit from above-typical doses of B6.

GABA is not well absorbed from the gut, so oral supplementation is often of little value. But carnosine, which stimulates GABA production, can be taken orally and absorbed well. Some data show carnosine as capable of improving anxiety and social attention in children with autism, at doses of 800 milligrams per day. In my own experience, children have shown a response with doses as low as 50 milligrams per day. With any of these tools, strive to work with a licensed provider whom you trust, who knows your child well, and who is open and curious to new solutions that can reduce the need for medications (and their unwanted side effects) while creating even bigger gains. Note that amino acids, when used individually and therapeutically, are best absorbed on an empty stomach when other proteins and amino acids are not in competition.

PRECAUTIONS FOR USING AMINO ACIDS

Amino acids have many roles in neurochemistry. If your child has any serious condition, such as an autoimmune condition, kidney or liver condition, seizure disorder, or thyroid condition, discuss your questions about using amino acids with your doctor before diving in. Children on psychiatric or seizure medications should have approval from their prescriber before using amino acids therapeutically. While these are ordinary compounds that occur in foods, taking them as a bolus or high dose can possibly interact with your child's medication. Most notable is using 5-hydroxytryptophan (5-HTP), which should not be mixed with SSRIs, unless your prescriber approves and guides you. Glutamine and aspartate may interfere with seizure medications. Some need nutrient cofactors to work correctly, as is true when using dimethylglycine (DMG). Children sometimes do poorly on this alone, but very well when folinic acid is added with it. Amino acids (supplements below ending in "–ine") work quickly. If you have approval from your prescriber, give them on an empty stomach so there are not competing amino acids for entry into cells. If you notice no change within three or four days of trying one, slowly increase the dose. If you notice a sudden negative change, withdraw the substance, and symptoms will resolve quickly. Some are best dosed in the morning, some at bedtime. For example, children with anxiety and apprehension about school may do poorly when 5-HTP is given in the morning, when cortisol is usually at its highest. Cortisol is a chemical we make as a natural response to stress, and otherwise for normal alertness. It is typically high as we are waking up, and lower later in the day and at bedtime. Boosting serotonin when cortisol is naturally at its apex may heighten anxiety rather than lower it for some children. Giving the same dose of 5-HTP late in the day may work much better, when it will aid sleep (it is a melatonin precursor) and lift mood, at a time of day when less cortisol is circulating.

ADRENAL FATIGUE

Adrenal glands sit atop our kidneys and are primarily responsible for stress response. As any parent of a child with autism or sensory integration disorder knows, stress, fear, anxiety, or outright terror are too common in the lives of these children. Insignificant events that a typical child would not register—a barking dog, the sudden sound of a glass breaking, a smoke alarm, even singing "Happy Birthday"—can pitch a child into trauma, tears, fight or flight, or frozen, blank-stare panic. Responding this way day in and day out to harmless occurrences exhausts and depletes the adrenal glands, which can in turn eventually disrupt sleep patterns, trigger depression, and leave your child disengaged and lethargic. Frequent illness and chronic fungal infection can cause adrenal fatigue as well. The extreme of adrenal fatigue is Addison's disease, in which the adrenal glands no longer produce enough cortisol. Cortisol helps maintain normal blood pressure, inflammatory responses, metabolism of foods, and a normal sense of alertness and well-being. For children with anxiety, supporting adrenal glands can be helpful, and there are gentle herbs for this purpose. Talk to a licensed naturopathic doctor (ND) about these herbs if you would like to use them. Generally safe introductory herbs are suggested below (licorice, ashwagandha, holy basil, and rhodiola rosea). Do not use all of them at once. If you want to try one, use it alone and do not mix it with other herbs on your own. If you have more questions or would like to combine them, talk to a licensed naturopath experienced in working with children. Homeopathic remedies treat episodes of panic well, but are not effective when used as a preventive. If your child is experiencing panic or extreme apprehension about a benign situation, and you know there is no underlying physical concern, Aconite is a remedy to consider. Aconite treats a sense of dread or terror, and signs of a panic attack: palpitations, sweating, blank stare, immobility due to terror, or a belief that death or danger is imminent. 12C or 30C pellets of Aconite, given every twenty minutes until resolved, can be effective. Stop using any homeopathic remedy once symptoms improve. More remedy is not better. It can be used like aspirin: Take it when a headache occurs; stop when the headache stops. Another dose is indicated only when symptoms stop improving.

ANOTHER NOTE. Cod liver oil and fish oil can have different therapeutic roles. Cod liver oil has vitamins A and D in it, while fish oil does not. Note the different applications of the two in the list below. EPA is the omega-3 fatty acid eicsapentanoic acid—which has shown some clinical effectiveness for mood and bipolar presentation. DHA is docohexaenoic acid, regarded as useful for attention and focus. DRI refers to Daily Recommended Intakes, which are set by the Food and Nutrition Board of the Institute of Medicine based on population data derived from healthy, typical children. That is, DRI are levels of nutrients recommended by the Food and Nutrition Board to maintain health in children with no heightened nutrient needs. Grams are noted with g, milligrams with mg, and micrograms with ug. Doses are per day unless otherwise stated.

Lastly, of course, do not use every recommendation below at once, and review your plans with your licensed health care provider. Use one at a time and go slowly. Withdraw it if there is a negative response. If you would like to start combining tools, engage a knowledgeable, licensed health care provider to help you and check on the Web for other parents' experiences and advice. Some sites, such as Revolution Health.com, post unbiased user reviews of supplements, herbs, and medications and list provider resources.

PROBLEM	TREATMENTS TO TRY	DISCUSS WITH YOUR PROVIDER
Anxiety/OCD	Replenish adequate calories	
	Replace inflammatory foods	
	Taurine, 200–1000 mg	
	Theanine, to 100–500 mg	
	Carnosine, to 100 mg	Carnosine in higher doses
	GABA, 500–1000 mg	Topical GABA
	Magnesium, to 300 mg	Magnesium in higher doses
	Epsom salts nightly with lavender	
	Chamomile, passion flower tinctures	
	NAC, single trial, 200–500 mg	NAC ongoing, >500 mg
		Rule out and treat Candida or dysbiosis
	Holy basil, to 300 mg, a.m.	
	Ashwaghanda, to 500 mg	
	Rhodiola rosea, to 100 mg	Rhodiola rosea >100 mg
Depression	Fish oil, to 1 tbsp	Cod liver oil, 1 tbsp or more
	5-HTP, 25–50 mg	5-HTP in higher doses or with SSRIs
	High-potency B group	
	Tyrosine, to 100 mg, a.m.	Tyrosine in higher doses
	Rhodiola rosea, to 100 mg	Rhodiola rosea >100 mg
	Replenish minerals to DRI	
Mood swings/bipolar	Adequate total calories	Rule out and treat Candida or dysbiosis
	EPA, 2–3 g	EPA >3 g
		Any use of SAM-e*
	Chromium to DRI	Chromium above DRI
	Tyrosine, 50–100 mg	Tyrosine >100 mg

Use St. John's Wort and 5-HTP with professional guidance in bipolar disorder.

PROBLEM	TREATMENTS TO TRY	DISCUSS WITH YOUR PROVIDER
Tactile hypersensitivity	Cod liver oil, 2 tsp	Cod liver oil >1 tbsp
	DHA, to 400 mg	
	Magnesium, to 300 mg	
	Full DRI for essential minerals	
Auditory sensitivity	High-potency probiotics	Rule out and treat Candida or dysbiosis
	B6, P5P, to double DRI	Higher doses of B6, P5P
	Magnesium, to 300 mg	Higher doses of magnesium
	Cod liver oil, to 2 tsp	Cod liver oil >1 tbsp
	Vitamin E, to 100 IU	Vitamin E >150IU
	NAC, 200–500 mg	NAC, ongoing, 500–1500 mg
	Carnosine, to 100 mg	Carnosine in higher doses
	Withdraw inflammatory foods	

PROBLEM	TREATMENTS TO TRY	DISCUSS WITH YOUR PROVIDER
Language/speech	Remove dietary opiates Replenish adequate calories Carnosine, to 100–200 mg DMG, TMG, B6, Mg† Methylcobalamin (B12) spray	Rule out and treat gut dysbiosis Higher doses of carnosine Methylcobalamin (B12) injection protocol
Motor skills/praxis	Replenish total calories Replenish minerals, especially magnesium Fish oil, to 1 tbsp Vitamin E, to double DRI	Rule out and chelate heavy metals
Eye contact	Cis-palmitate, in cod liver oil, 2 tsp Vitamin E, to double DRI Remove dietary opiates	Cis-palmitate >4000 IU Vitamin E >300 IU
Hyperactivity	Replenish minerals, especially sulfur DHA, 500–800 mg DMG, 100–500 mg, with folinic acid, to 800 ug	Rule out and treat gut dysbiosis
Attention/focus	Replenish adequate calories DHA, to 500 mg Full-potency B group Replenish all essential minerals (especially chromium, zinc, and magnesium) High-value protein breakfast	Methylcobalamin (B12) protocol, injected or inhaled Assure adequate iron status‡ Rule out and treat Candida or gut dysbiosis
Insomnia	Melatonin, 1–2 mg, p.m. 5-HTP, 25–50 mg, afternoon Taurine, to 500 mg, p.m. Theanine, to 100 mg, p.m. Epsom salts in bath, p.m. Magnesium, to 300 mg, p.m. (give with calcium) Sleepy Nights herb tincture, by WishGarden Passion flower or chamomile herb tinctures	Melatonin, >3 mg 5-HTP >50 mg Magnesium >300 mg
Toxicity		Treat Candida or dysbiosis Assess and treat heavy metals

PROBLEM	TREATMENTS TO TRY	DISCUSS WITH YOUR PROVIDER
	Liposomal Glutathione, 200–800 mg	
		Consider methylation support
Inflammation	Replace inflammatory foods Fish oils, to 2–3 g High-potency probiotics Replenish sulfur (Epsom salt baths) Replenish minerals to DRI Trial Splash if >4 major proteins are highly inflammatory	Treat Candida or dysbiosis
Social reciprocity	Replenish adequate calories Replenish minerals, to DRI High-potency B group DMG or TMG NAC, to 500 mg Cod liver oil, to 2 tsp Vitamin E, to 100 IU Carnosine, 100–200 mg, a.m. Methyl-B12 sublingual spray	Treat Candida or dysbiosis Assess and treat heavy metals NAC >500 mg Carnosine >200 mg Methyl-B12 nasal spray or injection
Weak, picky appetite	Replenish minerals, to DRI Zinc, to 30 mg Replace inflammatory foods High-potency probiotics Avoid vitamin A >3000 IU Trial Splash	 Rule out antigliadin antibody Treat Candida or dysbiosis Consider meds to increase appetite (e.g., Periactin)

*S-adenosyl methionine (SAM-e): Use with professional guidance and caution in manic disorders, bipolar disorder, and ADHD.

†DMG is dimethylglycine; TMG is trimethylglycine. These are methyl donors. When used with a full complement of the B group, high-dose B6, and magnesium, some children show gains in expressive language.

‡Poor iron status in children has been linked to math learning disabilities and other cognitive deficits.

Micronutrients Relative to Signs and Symptoms

VITAMIN/MINERAL	DEFICIENCY SIGNS
Thiamin	Confusion Peripheral paralysis Weakness, wasting

VITAMIN/MINERAL	DEFICIENCY SIGNS
	Loss of ankle and knee jerk reflexes Painful calf muscles Irritability, listlessness
Riboflavin	Dermatitis around nose and lips Cracking at corners of mouth Hypersensitivity to light Reddening of cornea Magenta tongue
Niacin	Smooth tongue surface, swollen tongue Irritability, listlessness
B6 (pyridoxine)	Dermatitis Cracks at corners of mouth Irritated sweat glands Smooth tongue Seizures Irritability, listlessness
Folacin	Smooth, swollen, or cracked tongue Diarrhea, loss of villi and their enzymes Fatigue, depression, confusion Megaloblastic anemia, suppressed immune function
Vitamin B12	Smooth, swollen, cracked tongue Pernicious or megaloblastic anemia Tactile hypersensitivity Loss of vibratory or position sense (vestibular sense)
Pantothenic acid	Vomiting, irritable bowel Insomnia, fatigue, listlessness "Burning feet" sensation
Biotin	Scaly dry skin Hair loss Depression, lassitude Muscle pains Anorexia or nausea
Zinc excess	Metallic taste in mouth Nausea/vomiting
Zinc deficit	Poor appetite Poor growth Patchy dermatitis, hair loss Slow wound healing Impaired sense of smell/taste White dots on nails Delayed sexual maturation

VITAMIN/MINERAL	DEFICIENCY SIGNS
Copper excess	Tremors, liver inflammation, difficulty speaking/swallowing Involuntary jerky movement Gold-green rings at cornea
Copper deficit	Fatigue, bleeding under skin Anemia with low WBC count
Magnesium excess	Weakness, low blood pressure, palpitations
Magnesium deficit	Nausea, muscle weakness, irritability, derangement, high thirst, arrhythmia
Vitamin D deficit	Rickets, bone pain and weakness Muscle pain Hypothyroidism secondary to hypocalcemia or poor vitamin D status
Vitamin D excess	Thirst, weakness, anxiety High blood pressure, high calcium in blood
Vitamin A deficit	Night blindness, light sensitivity In ASD, lack of eye contact (cis-palmitate) Xeropthalmia, Bitot's spots Dry scaly skin Frequent infection Vitamin A absorption impeded by low-fat diet or fat malabsorption
Vitamin A excess	Cracked red lips, hair loss Low appetite, bone pain, headache
Vitamin E	Impaired reflexes, difficulty walking, weak muscles
Essential fatty acids	Skin rashes, dry scaly skin Excessive inflammatory responses Decreased skin pigmentation Poor sleep pattern Hostile or aggressive behavior Inattention Tantrums

Final Thoughts on Supplements

Use these judiciously—that is, only continue with supplements that have a clear benefit. Expect the need for supplements to change as your child grows and changes. Most important, your child needs food more than he needs supplements. We all would like that one magic medication or supplement, but children with autism, ADHD, sensory integration disorder, or challenges for mood, anxiety, learning, or behavior usually have multiple nutrition problems, and varied needs biochemically and physiologically. If there was one solid fix, we'd have found it by now, and every child who needed it would be using it. Supplements can help overcome problems with absorption, toxicity, inflammation, or poor diets. Regard them as repairs or supports that your child may need for a while, but not forever. The long-term goal of nutrition care is typical absorption and tolerance for an unrestricted diet. When a gut is working entirely as it is meant to, supplements become less necessary, as do restricted diets. Therapeutic dosing for specific conditions can still be beneficial, but expect to refine and revisit your child's supplement protocol at least twice a year. Adverse events with supplements are by far rare, compared to adverse events from medications. They are relatively quite safe, and any negative effects will resolve in nearly every case with withdrawal of the supplement. If you have used a supplement for a long while that your child may no longer need, taper it off, as you would a medication. If removing it triggers a negative outcome, reintroduce it at a lower dose, and use only the dose you need to resolve the problem. As always, discuss concerns or questions with whomever on your team is most knowledgeable on therapeutic dosing of supplements. Most pediatricians are less familiar with using supplements. If this is true in your doctor's case, check with a licensed naturopathic doctor, or a DAN MD with several years' experience.

SIX

Shop, Cook, Eat

Making Nutrition Work in Your Kitchen

Special diets for children are therapeutic measures, equal and at times even greater in importance than a medication. After all the footwork is done to identify what your child might best eat, and to encourage a normal appetite and interest in food, what are you going to make for dinner? What goes in the lunch sack? What happens at the pizza party, when your child is not eating gluten? There are many great cookbooks for children on special diets, and the Internet abounds with recipe resources. When my editor said she wanted recipes, I wondered what I could possibly add to this existing body of information. Many parents have learned to enjoy pretty good eats in a household without gluten, casein, soy, junk, peanuts, walnuts, pecans, and even eggs—something my own family has survived, too. The following strategies have worked well:

- Consider making your entire kitchen at least partly compliant with your child's diet strategy. For example, stock and cook only gluten-free pasta, instead of boiling and serving two different types when you make a batch of spaghetti and meatballs.
- If there are siblings who are eating a regular diet, plan ahead on what will be told to whom about the special diet. Let important others know (grandparents, child care providers) so your children receive the same clear message from everyone.
- Older siblings may be ready to lend support or at least agree not to interfere, by helping you avoid transgressions into the wrong foods for the affected child.
- Younger ones may be able to eat the new foods without complaint, depending on their age and stage.
- Single-child or smaller families seem to have more success when the household complies with the new diet. For example, pull all wheat foods out of your kitchen, and stock only gluten-free flours, cookies, breads, pastas and so on for everyone.

In practice, I have not yet encountered a child who didn't notice when there were different foods around the table, no matter what the diagnosis. For family meals, it works best to simply serve everyone the same items. It is, of course, easier for the cook, but it also eliminates strife at the table. In our era of endless consumer choice, it is fine for siblings to make a sacrifice at a meal a couple times a week to include another with special needs. One strategy is to allow siblings on regular diets to enjoy their favorite foods at other times—parties, lunches, schools, breakfasts, snacks—but for sit-down family meals—and you should have them if at all possible on a regular basis, at least two or three times a week—serve everyone a meal that complies with your special-needs child's restrictions. More than a convenient way to manage menus, this is an invaluable expression of love and inclusion.

What to Tell Your Child

All children are different. First and foremost, work with a strategy that suits your child's needs, based on information in this book. Next, review these thoughts about your child's age and stage:

- **Infants (age 0–12 months):** Of course, an infant needs love, nourishment, joy, attachment to his parents, and a safe, clean home. Infants will pick up quickly on parents' anxiety and they need to hear nothing of their own health foibles. If you have an infant who needs diet interventions very early, strategize with your pediatrician about it, and find good supports outside your home to help you manage anxieties about your child's progress and health. Look for postpartum support groups where it is safe to share how you really feel, or find trusted friends and family to encourage you, let you catch some sleep, and give you time away from the baby. This way, you can focus your caretaking energies for the baby in a positive, calm way, while meeting your own care needs, too.

- **Toddlers (age 1–3 years):** You are fully in charge. Don't explain, don't complain. Simply begin making the switches you choose. If your toddler has reflux, chronic loose stool, and a picky poor appetite, simpler carbs from the SCD list will be easier to digest. Allow gluten-free treats (breads, pasta, cookies, bars, fruit breads), because small children need these calories, and they need them as carbohydrates. As always, correcting bowel flora will help your child digest these foods more normally. If there are unresolved and significant GI symptoms, a capsule endoscopy is the ultimate tool to tell you what is going on. A pill-size camera takes pictures of the intestine as it passes through the GI tract.

- **School age (4–12 years):** M Depending on your child's abilities, explain as little or as much as you feel is appropriate about new foods. Whenever it is reasonable for her to participate and choose, let her. For example: "We are using new foods so you can grow up healthy, strong, and happy. Everyone is different. Some people can eat everything, some people avoid foods that bother them. Do you want to try the pastas first, or should we try a cake?" Or: "We are going to see if a gluten-free diet helps you feel more relaxed, focused, and energetic. We will try it for four months. Let's shop for cookbooks online. Which one looks good?"

- **Teens (13–18):** Low-functioning teens with autism need brief, concrete information. You will be choosing what foods to start with, based on your own ability to best meet the challenge. More adult than child, this age group's behaviors during opiate withdrawal can be fierce. Still, they are no less deserving of the opportunity to resolve painful GI symptoms or function better than any other child of any age. Engage your provider and support network and make a plan of how to contain spikes in behavior, if they occur. Discuss with your provider the use of encapsulated charcoal, a tool that absorbs toxins in the gut to help them be harmlessly excreted. Choose a probiotic that effectively binds opiate compounds and oxalates in the gut (MindLinx or VSL3 are examples of probiotics that have shown effectiveness for these tasks).

- **If your child is in residential care:** Care plans in any clinical setting are driven by found problems. It won't work to simply ask to implement a special diet. Providers working with your child have to find the problems and document them first. A special diet in a residential setting requires the full support of the care team, with coordination and leadership from the primary authorizing physician at your child's facility. Kitchen staff who serve a number of individuals will be asked to make special foods for your child, and they, of course, only take orders from the dietitian and the doctors in charge, not you. Arrange a meeting and ask your child's primary provider how this could best be approached. A gastroenterology consult may help. Request ELISA testing, celiac screen, antigliadin antibody test, and stool culture. Work with those results and make a plan together. This may also profoundly change what doses or types of medications your child needs, so you will want to include that prescriber in the process at some point.

The suggestions that follow for shopping, cooking, and eating are not intended to expound on the benefits of any one diet over another, but are simply a means to begin what may seem like an overwhelming task. Gluten-free foods are an easy place to start. They are widely available and easy to let your child try.

Shop

The worst part of all this is invariably the beginning, when parents groan with dread about changing food shopping routines. Shopping for a family and preparing food are not usually at the top of anyone's list of favorite activities, and cheers to you if they are. Rearranging how you get what you need in the kitchen has a learning curve, so give yourself time for it. Take consolation in the fact that this is much easier than it was even just five years ago, and that the foods you will need are everywhere now. Most better supermarkets are aware of special diet needs by now, and are stocking plenty of gluten- and casein-free foods, which permits you to continue shopping where you usually do for the most part. Megamarkets such as Trader Joe's, Whole Foods (which lists more than a thousand gluten-free items on its website), and Wild Oats offer most of what you'll need, and most bigger population centers have their local favorite health food stores, too. You can buy these specialty foods on the Internet, from gluten-free bread to organic buffalo meat. My household receives a monthly shipment directly from a gluten-free bakery for sandwich bread, doughnuts, and English muffins. We bake fresh rolls and breadsticks with a mix (Chébé, from Vermont), buy specialty items as we like (scones, piecrusts, or muffins from Whole Foods), or create pizza crusts from a recipe. We avoid dairy ingredients in these items and substitute accordingly when baking.

Knowing a bit about gluten-free flours is a good idea. If you enjoy baking, an excellent resource is Rebecca Reilly's *Gluten Free Baking*. Besides recipes, there is a useful breakdown in this book of what gluten-free dry ingredients will work in your pantry, plus explanations of which flours work best for what. Bean flours have a stronger flavor that suits piecrusts; sweet rice flour is stickier and keeps gluten-free baked goods moister. Most recipes call for combinations of flours to make them work well. Here are the flour options: brown rice flour, sweet rice flour, white rice flour, bean flours, arrowroot, chickpea flour, cornmeal and corn flour, garfava flour (part garbanzo bean flour and part chickpea flour), potato flour, potato starch, quinoa flour, soy flour, and tapioca starch. Xanthan gum is used often in gluten-free baking since it gives a leavening boost, a job otherwise filled by gluten.

Allow for a Gradual Transition

Don't buy everything on your first special diet shopping spree. Now that there is so much food out there that suits these diets, it's easy to enthusiastically shop for everything GFCF, only to have most of it rejected by your child. As kids try a nibble of one thing after another then toss it across the room, a lot of the expensive stuff you just bought will spoil while it waits in the fridge or cupboard for a more favorable review. So buy just a few items to start. It will take some experimenting to see which ones your child likes better than others. For example, if your child likes to eat pancakes for breakfast, start with a gluten-free mix and make it with almond milk. Say nothing. If he balks, you should shrug, admit nothing, and give him his favorite again the next day. In a few days, try another product. You will eventually find one he likes. If push comes to shove, you can use my mother's sage advice: Don't explain, don't complain (especially to a kid). You can say, "We can't buy that other kind anymore. Let's put apple juice and cinnamon in the new recipe. You can be the first reviewer of this new kind of pancake, so let's invent one you love." Another good thing about gradually transitioning this way is that, though it takes longer, it will be less stressful and disruptive for your child. Nonverbal children with autism will only be able to show disapproval with action. Continue to offer fluid calories if they downright refuse the new foods, and remain calm. Make sure the bowel flora piece is well treated, and the acceptance of new items will usually go faster.

Pulling out dietary sources of opiate compounds and treating gut dysbiosis creates quite a physiological rearrangement for anyone. Some parents and providers advocate the fire hose approach, where you simply blast these things out as fast as possible to rescue a child deep in the autism abyss. Others choose to work more methodically and gradually. My preference? Depends on the family, and the parents. Unless a parent is particularly stalwart, and can withstand the furies that ensue with the fire hose approach, I have observed that a gradual approach seems to be more successful, simply because it is easier for both parent and child to comply. As always, trust your own instincts about what suits you, because you are in charge, and you are responsible for carrying out the care plan.

More examples of items to ease into:

- If toaster waffles are a morning favorite, switch in GF buckwheat frozen toaster waffles (my preference) or Van's GF waffles. These are in the freezer case of many supermarkets now, and are reliably available at Whole Foods or Trader Joe's. You can drizzle with flax oil, berries, or applesauce. If that goes well, move on to the next item.

- If your child eats Goldfish crackers every day for a snack, substitute Tings (corn puffs that taste like cheese puffs), GF pretzels (Glutino or Ener-G brands are excellent), or corn tortilla chips. Or take a leap of faith and give something healthier, such as macadamia nuts with a few sunflower seeds and semisweet chocolate chips (this might be too much too fast for a Goldfish-addicted kid).

- If pasta is a staple, check out Tinkyada brand gluten-free rice pastas. These are available in every shape, and are usually well accepted by children; others made with bean, quinoa, or corn flours are allowable but their taste and texture are sometimes too different for kids accustomed to wheat. Follow the cooking instructions carefully, and err on the side of undercooking. Overcooked rice pasta disintegrates fast. I have found that at altitude, where I live, I need to cook this pasta two to three minutes less than the package instructs.

Withdraw the Lesser Opiate First

As mentioned in Chapter 4, it often works well to withdraw your child's "lesser opiate" first, that is, the one she doesn't favor or eat as often. For milk-addicted children, this means quietly substituting gluten-free foods while continuing to allow dairy at first. Completely replace all the gluten, then tackle the dairy. You might notice your child gradually refusing the new gluten-free foods because she leans harder on that dairy-sourced opiate. This phase will pass and improve as soon as you pull out the dairy protein. For kids who love bread, pasta, starchy stuff, and pizza above all else, it means yanking the dairy stuff first.

Since your demeanor around the special diet intervention and new foods has a big impact on how your child will accept all the changes, choose the strategy you are most comfortable with. Gluten-free foods are easy to plug into special diets since they are now widely available and often so resemble their wheat counterparts that children do not notice the difference, until the opiate withdrawal phase hits. The most difficult thing to mimic is a good crusty baguette, or something like a puffy doughnut. Serviceable gluten-free versions exist, but they can't achieve the texture we all love in the real thing. After all, gluten is exactly what makes dough springy, stretchy, soft, and delicate all at once. Other grains can't do that, so tools such as eggs, egg whites, xanthan gum, and baking powder are pressed harder into service to improve the texture when you bake your own items. See the list of gluten-free cookbooks and sites in this chapter for recipes and tricks that make gluten-free foods taste good, so that the opiate transition is eased.

Sources for Gluten-Free Foods

Many manufacturers now make gluten-free foods, and some are devoted to gluten-free processing entirely. The way to know the difference is simply to read labels. Gluten-free means gluten-free. "Wheat-free" does not mean gluten-free, because other ingredients besides wheat contain gluten, such as barley, barley malt, malt, oats, and rye. In addition, modified food starch is usually made from wheat flour, unless it is otherwise specified as starch from corn, tapioca, or potato. However, because it is not actual wheat, a label can still proclaim the product is "wheat-free." Individuals who are extremely sensitive to gluten, as are persons with true celiac disease, should often avoid processed foods with caramel color, soy sauce, vinegar, or unspecified flavorings and thickeners. Some vinegars and anything containing these vinegars contain gluten; malt and balsamic vinegars certainly will. At the start of a GF diet, do your best to avoid these trace sources of gluten. Later, excepting true celiac patients, children seem to tolerate these gluten minutiae better, leaving you to focus on the major food sources of wheat (if they still don't after a year or more gluten-free, perhaps something is missing from your treatment plan). Wheat flour, wheat starch, food starch, or modified food starch is often used to thicken commercial and restaurant soups, dressings, gravies, and sauces. Corn starch, tapioca starch, and potato starch also thicken these foods well, so there is nothing imperative about using wheat for this.

What about cross-contamination? In our litigious culture, food manufacturers are obligated to tell you if a product may have traces of an allergen. Generally, I encourage parents to focus energies on larger problems, rather than expecting to eliminate all likelihood of ever encountering an allergen contaminant. Obviously, children with life-threatening allergies must be this careful, but those with lesser consequences from offending foods do not need to be this careful, in my opinion. You might request that your GF pasta in a restaurant be boiled in a separate pot from the one used for wheat pasta. But nano-amounts of cross-contamination are relevant only for people who have life-threatening anaphylaxis to a food or supersensitive celiac, not the possibility of forming a few opiates. In a perfect world, children using diet restrictions to avoid opiate formation would never see a molecule of gluten, casein, or soy. But the burden of anxiety and stress this can impart to a household or a child outweighs its benefit much of the time. If your child is so sensitive that such a small trace triggers a big behavioral reaction, especially after six months or more of using the restriction, something is missing from your care plan. Recovery should be progressing such that a speck of gluten from caramel coloring can go unnoticed by your child's liver, brain, and GI tract. Talk with your provider about assessing digestive enzyme output, or adding enzymes specific to these proteins. Make sure micronutrients that assist the function of these enzymes are on board (especially biotin, B vitamins, and minerals such as zinc or magnesium). Lastly, consider assessing heavy metals, since these will disable many enzymes in the body. Gluten and casein can pop up in anything from toothpaste to medications, flavorings, and chewable vitamins. Avoid these obvious sources, too, along with foods containing them, but leave room for your child to feel as unfettered as possible. Fretting over whether the Play-Doh is gluten-free won't make or break your child's nutrition intervention, unless he handles it and eats it daily. If he is literally eating Play-Doh daily, this is indicative of pica and an opiate kick from it. Obviously, you need to give your child something else to play with, because he shouldn't be eating gluten-free Play-Doh daily either!

Look for these gluten-free resources, brands, and prepared foods:

Amy's brand prepared foods and meals	www.Amys.com
Bob's Red Mill baking mixes	www.BobsRedMill.com
Kinnikinnick breads, bagels, doughnuts, and more	www.Kinnikinnick.com
Tinkyada pasta	www.Tinkyada.com
Whole Foods Gluten Free Bakehouse	www.WholeFoodsMarket.com
Ener-G snacks, breads, and mixes	www.Ener-G.com
Chebe mixes for rolls, calzones, breadsticks	www.Chebe.com
Pancake and cake mixes	www.AuthenticFoods.com
Pamela's cookies, baking mixes, and flavorings	www.PamelasProducts.com

More, More, and Even More

www.celiac.com	www.gfmeals.com
www.gfcfdiet.com	www.glutenfree.com
www.gfcfgourmet.com	www.glutenfreeforum.com
www.gflinks.com	www.glutenfreeinfo.com
www.gfmall.com	www.livingwithout.com

Adding the Casein Restriction to Your Shopping List

This, too, is relatively easy, but for the opposite reason that clearing out the gluten is simple: Frankly, there are no great substitutes for cheese. You will mostly be removing cheese from your child's diet and replacing it with new foods entirely. Aside from cheese, casein is in all fluid cow's milk and subsequent products, including lactose-free milk, puddings, creamy dressings and soups, and many baked goods and snack foods. It is also in butter. Let's start with what to buy in place of cheese.

Some cheese facsimiles are available, and these are made from soy or rice typically. They don't melt right, and they taste weird—just my frank opinion. Others contain casein but can be called "dairy-free" because there is no actual intact cheese or milk in them. Some children take to them, but most leave cheese behind in lieu of new horizons as their appetites broaden with recovery. See options at GalaxyFoods.com. Ultimately, after some gut healing has been secured, reintroduction of organic goat cheeses is sometimes reasonable, with the use of digestive enzymes that target gluten and casein peptides, and with probiotics that do the same. One thing that makes cheese so good is the dairy fat in it. Subbing in similar textures can work. Here are some ways around cheese:

Pizza or Calzones

Make your own gluten-free (buy crust ready-made, or make your own, or buy Amy's ready-to-bake GF pizza with soy cheese, or try Chébé mixes for calzones) and top with caramelized onion (white onion sautéed in ghee or CF margarine and brown sugar), sliced olives, pepperoni, and/or thin-sliced green, red, or orange pepper. Peppers have a sweetness that emerges with broiling or baking that kids can take to in many cases. Put your own barbecued chicken leftovers in a calzone with mayo, minced scallion, and cilantro.

Grilled Cheese

Experiment with the cheese substitutes. If that's a flop, try grilled chicken salad or grilled ham salad sandwiches. For kids with texture aversions, use a food processor to finely grind chicken or ham. For chicken, add dill, salt, pepper, minced celery leaf, minced fresh basil, and mayonnaise. For ham salad, add a few drops of dill pickle juice, dill spice, and mayonnaise. The classic accompaniment for kids— tomato soup—is available ready to heat and eat from Imagine or Pacific Foods, gluten- and casein-free.

MAC AND CHEESE

A few companies have put out GFCF versions of this staple for wheat-and-dairy-addicted kids, which are worth a try. A better scenario is bringing your child's interest in new foods forward to the point that mac and cheese is a meal that is almost forgotten. Try salads with elbow, spiral, or penne pasta, olive oil, sliced olives, minced prosciutto, cilantro, green peas, wax beans, or any other favorites mixed in. Lots of garlic is often appreciated, with salt, cracked pepper, and even a little turmeric for coloring.

YOGURT

Soy yogurts are available, but for children avoiding dietary opiates, these should not become a daily staple. If this soft food is a comforting favorite for your child and you must find a similar replacement, you might try tapioca pudding or egg custards made with equal parts almond milk and coconut milk. Some children do fine avoiding cow yogurt and subbing in goat yogurt, but this will have the potential for forming an opiate also. Use digestive enzymes and probiotics that degrade gluten and casein peptides if your child is eating these foods.

GOLDFISH CRACKERS

These are eaten by the cupful, daily, by many a wheat- or dairy-addicted kid. They are full of cheddar cheese, which is yummy, but to be avoided on the casein restriction. Other cheese crackers must go, too. For kids who need the crunch and the salt fix (don't worry, this, too, can pass), sub in Glutino or Ener-G pretzels, onion rice crackers, Blue Diamond Nut Thins, tortilla chips or corn chips, or Tings corn puffs. Gluten-free cereals are fine to munch on dry as well. Your child can be expected to progress to more nutritious options like a trail mix eventually, with dried fruits, macadamia nuts, cashews, sunflower seeds, and dark chocolate chips. These foods are high oxalate, so kids who struggle with oxalates may have to stick to the processed snack items until they have balanced a leaky gut situation, high yeast, marginal vitamin K status, or calcium absorption.

PUDDING

If your child loves to carry pudding cups to school, sub in rice-based pudding cups, Jell-O cups, applesauce (experiment with different flavors), or even a homemade tapioca or coconut custard. Yes, some of this is junk food, but so are those dairy-based pudding cups. Eventually, you can work on healthier alternatives if you like, but in the meantime, you will be giving your child a version that is actually preferable.

PUMPKIN PIE

This gets special mention because many families would not have Thanksgiving without it. Gluten-free crusts finally worked for me with a recipe from Rebecca Reilly's book, *Gluten Free Baking*. For the pumpkin custard, a foray into soy milk is acceptable since this is such a special occasion. Replace evaporated milk with WestSoy Vanilla Soy Shake, Silk Vanilla Soy Milk, or Silk Vanilla Soy Creamer. The vanilla soy milks are sweet, so adjust the sugar in the recipe downward to taste. Plain soy milk can be used, too, though the thicker consistency of the flavored, sweetened soy milk works better for this application. If that is simply verboten, almond milk or hazelnut milk would be the next choice. Without thickeners worked into the recipe, rice or potato milk may be too watery for the desired result, but worth a try for those avoiding nuts or oxalates.

BUTTER

Use ghee, which is clarified butter (all dairy solids including protein have been removed), as much as you like. It is expensive, but allowable. For baking where a stiffer texture is needed, as in a piecrust, ghee can work well. For a softer texture, as for a big chewy cookie, margarine is acceptable. Earth Balance margarine is casein-free, and also free of trans fats and hydrogenated fats.

FLUID COW'S MILK

Since even small amounts can be so disruptive for children with evidence of opiates, allergy, or intolerance, cow's milk becomes more harm than good in these cases and needs to be withdrawn. Children who have shown high urine casein-sourced "opiates" will benefit most if they completely avoid it, and all other casein sources. Unlike a low-fat diet, where a little fat is not only okay but necessary, a casein-free diet should be casein-free to be effective, because each dose of "a little" casein will elicit dozens of opiate-like peptides for the brain—enough to impede progress for language, behavior, sleep, or cognition. Kids with some inflammation from this protein (but no opiate formation) tend to benefit with less irritability, improved asthma symptoms, normalization of stools, and improved sensory regulation as they reduce or eliminate casein. Exactly how much casein in the diet they can handle, if any, is best discovered by completely removing it at first for two to four months, then adding back a small amount to see how it goes. If all seems fine, track your child's functional and behavioral progress; antibodies to food proteins are dose-responsive. If after a month of re-exposure you have seen no negative shifts, your child is showing improved tolerance and may continue.

Younger children still drinking a lot of milk need substitutes that are nutritionally equivalent. Milks from rice, potato, nuts, or hemp do not fill the bill and should not be used as a primary protein or calorie source. If your child loves them, offer servings of a high-value protein that she will reliably eat every time, three times a day: egg, all-natural hot dog, meat, chicken (try Bell & Evans gluten-free chicken tenders or nuggets), chili with ground beef, turkey. If something like this is eaten often, then the low-value milks are allowable up to three cups per day. If your child refuses solids that give high-value protein and only accepts fluid calories, then you will need to add protein to the milk substitutes. Use medical foods such as Ultracare for Kids, or amino acid supplements such as AminoPlex. Powders made from whey and soy are not allowable on the casein restriction. Powders from egg are available but can be difficult to dissolve. You will need to deliver roughly 25–30 grams of protein from these daily, so that is several spoonfuls of supplemental powder. Boost calories with coconut milk, and add fresh fruits if your child likes those flavors. If none of this works, look to Pepdite or Splash as a fluid milk substitute. Alternative milks are fine for substitutions in some recipes calling for milk, such as pancakes, cookies, or most baked goods. When a recipe calls for a thick, high-fat milk such as condensed milk or cream, this is an occasion when a soy milk might work best, such as Silk Soy Creamers. These are made with tapioca starch to give them the thicker consistency we love in cream. Rice milk or almond milk may leave your recipe too watery.

CREAMY DRESSINGS

Ranch dressing a favorite? Your child might like creamy lime dressing instead, which relies on eggs to achieve the same texture of a ranch dressing. See the recipe later in this chapter. Use the basic procedure of this recipe to experiment with other flavors. You can also easily make your own mayonnaise blend as a base for any creamy dressing (recipes are readily available on the Web and in many cookbooks).

EGGNOG

This Christmastime favorite has all the heart-unhealthy ingredients: heavy cream and lots of eggs, not to mention lots of bourbon, dark rum, sugar, nutmeg, and a block of premium vanilla ice cream to float in the punch bowl. For kids with special needs, all those calories and fats can sometimes be helpful. You can make a festive and suitable alternative version without casein (or alcohol!) that lets kids feel like they are getting a supreme treat. See the recipe later in this chapter.

Casein-Free Alternative Foods

www.GalaxyFoods.com	For cheese substitutes
www.ImagineFoods.com	For frozen treats, nut or rice milks, and soups
www.earthbalance.net/product.html	For casein-free margarine (no trans or hydrogenated fats)
www.SilkSoyMilk.com	For special-occasion baking, try Silk Soy Creamers
www.PacificFoods.com	For alternative milks, prepared soups, gluten-free gravies

Cooking Strategies: It's Easier Than You Think

Think in terms of what you usually like to cook and serve for your family, and adapt it. This is what you will actually be doing, rather than completely pitching what you already do well. There is no need to yank all your family's favorites off the table, or ostracize a special-needs child further by giving her a separate plate of food every night. Check your favorite cookbooks that have nothing to do with dietary restrictions, for recipes you'd like to continue using; they can probably be converted to compliance with a special diet. Recipes that must have butter can succeed with ghee or CF margarine (butter has casein and whey solids in it and is withdrawn on a casein restriction). You can also use oils and reduce other liquids in a recipe that calls for butter. For milk, try rotating in milk alternatives or even fruit juice, if you're making a pancake, waffle, or muffin. For thickeners in a sauce or gravy try using starch from tapioca, corn, or potato, or rice flour, or splurge on ready-to-heat gluten-free gravy from the store. A trick that works very well for thickening sauces is to finely mince onion or garlic in about equal parts to the butter and starch. Sauté the onion or garlic for a bit first in the "butter" or olive oil (don't burn it), then add the starch. When you begin to add your liquid, it will thicken better.

Your family can still enjoy pasta dishes, grilled anything, barbecue (check your favorite store-bought sauce for gluten ingredients; gluten-free versions are available), many casseroles and stews, and basic meals that feature a meat, chicken, or acceptable fish (some have lower mercury content than others*). Besides the fact that pizza night will mean you are not buying it from your local favorite pizza parlor anymore (maybe it's a pizza party where you make your own), what may change are side items such as rolls, buns, or breadsticks. So what? Get to work with Chebe mixes or other resources for gluten-free versions. For breaded chicken or tempura, buy ready-made (Bell & Evans) gluten-free chicken tenders or nuggets, and mix up your own tempura batter (see the recipe later in this chapter, from Bette Hagman). Introduce yourself to side dishes such as cooked quinoa; variations on rice, risotto, or wild rice; rice salads; hearty vegetables such as acorn or butternut squash, beets, or snap peas; or salsas that use corn, beans, heirloom tomatoes, green beans, mango, peach—anything goes. Even instant mashed potatoes are serviceable with rice or almond milk, and ghee or CF margarine. Or use your own bakers and stuff with bacon, mushrooms, olive oil, avocado—whatever works.

Back to that pizza party. If part of the fun is that you're ordering in rather than cooking, look into your options. Franchises that offer gluten- and casein-free (or at least GFCF-diminished) selections are

*To eat fish or not? Some have lower mercury content than others. Some families avoid it altogether, while others allow servings judiciously. Visit www.cfsan.fda.gov/~frf/sea-mehg.html to judge for yourself.

popping up: Pei Wei Asian Diner, Chipotle Mexican Grill, Rumbi Island Grill, even Pizza Fusion offers items that are compliant or nearly compliant and that kids like. Traces of gluten or casein are preferable to eating a fully.loaded wheat and dairy pizza pie. You still get your night off, and your other kids might find something they like, too. Check www.gfmeals.com for more restaurant resources. And below you'll find some ideas for arranging your household's food day to day.

Meal Plans

BREAKFASTS

Gluten-free, nitrate/nitrite-free, MSG-free breakfast meats are not to be forgotten for kids on special diets. Sausage, bacon, or ham can be bought with wholesome ingredients. Gluten-free versions of starchy breakfast favorites are easy to find, from pancake mixes, to frozen waffles and cereals, to toast or scones. The bigger challenge may be getting some protein into your child in the morning. Along with breakfast meats or eggs, some children will accept a smoothie or shake with protein powder added. Use at least 5 grams of added protein if you take this approach; 10 to 20 grams are preferable, if your child will tolerate the texture of the powder to this degree. It is also entirely acceptable to reheat a favorite leftover and serve it for breakfast—a soup, a stew, fried rice with egg and vegetables, last night's chicken tenders, or whatever your child likes. Going out the door with something in the stomach is better than nothing for a child by far, so if your child eats only the starchy stuff to begin with, be patient and work with it—it will change eventually, if your total nutrition intervention is on track. If your child tolerates peanut butter, add it to toast or smoothies to up the calories, protein, and fat. If she does not, try using sesame tahini or other nut/seed butters in its place. For kids who like hot cereal, certified gluten-free oats are now available (though more expensive) from Bob's Red Mill or www.GlutenFreeOats.com. Adding flax oil, some maple syrup, unsweetened coconut milk, or sesame tahini imparts staying power to oatmeal or hot rice cereal, as do crushed nuts, raisins, bananas, or berries. Another likely favorite is "San Diego Roll Ups," named after what was served for breakfast at a DAN conference there years ago: soft warm corn tortillas, guacamole or ripe avocado slices, scrambled eggs, and mild salsa rolled up and eaten as finger food. Chopped sausage is good in these, too.

LUNCHES

For sandwich lovers, not much should change here. Use a bread such as Kinnikinnick's Gluten-Free Italian Sandwich Bread or their brown sandwich bread, and whatever favorite fillings your child already likes. Toasting gluten-free breads lightly before making the sandwich and packing it into the lunch box makes them taste better. If a cheese slice is de rigueur, this is where a substitute from a company such as Galaxy Foods might fit best. Some kids do well with a single-serving thermos carried to school, with a protein-and-calorie-rich item in it such as chili, stew, or GF elbow macaroni with meat sauce. Hearty rice or pasta salads, using GF corkscrew or penne pasta, can also work. I use green peas, fresh basil or cilantro, minced ham or chicken, sliced olives, garlic, and any homemade dressing. Vegetable sushi is not too far out either, once children start eating more adventurously. It is easy for them to carry, and you can buy it ready-made at many supermarkets now (you will need to sub in your own wheat-free tamari, which is soy sauce without wheat or gluten). Some sushi rice may have traces of gluten, and you can decide if that matters enough in your child's case. Soft corn tortilla roll-ups also work well when filled with chicken salad, turkey slices and lime dressing; or try a good-quality, additive-free hot dog, bratwurst, turkey dog, or chicken dog. Grill your hot dog on the stove top, then roll it in a warmed corn tortilla with any preferred condiment (mustard, relish, catsup). Place it back on the griddle to seal the tortilla.

There Is Plenty to Eat

There is no shortage of great food to buy, prepare, and eat for kids using special diets. While there will always be moments where your child isn't eating what his friends or siblings get to have, for the most part, there is little reason for him to feel slighted, left out, or singled out. The bigger obstacles parents usually bemoan are getting a picky eater to eat all this new stuff, and fearing intestinal yeast overgrowth if they give their child the right amount of food for his age and stage. As this book suggests often, correct the underlying problems that make eating and absorbing food painful, uncomfortable, or difficult, and your child's appetite will likely restore itself. If your child is not showing an improved, more varied appetite on his special diet, then something may be wrong. Rule out poor status for zinc and iron; check the dose of vitamin A or cod liver oil, and be sure it is below 4000 IU daily (too much will depress appetite). If reflux is in the way, make sure Candida or Clostridia are not present, and request the strongest allowable medications for these (typically, Diflucan and Flagyl). A full supplement holiday also helps sort through the mists. They may simply be irritating your child, who needs food more than supplements. Take a break for a week, and add back only the ones that are essential per your provider, or that trigger a clear benefit.

Classroom Strategies

Food is always popping up unannounced in school. This is one place where a special-diet child may be inadvertently left out. To avoid this, speak to the point person for your child. It might be the lead resource teacher, classroom teacher, your child's aid, or even the principal. Ask the school to store a cache of treats to use as incentives for work done, to share as your child likes, and enjoy during special occasions when food comes out. Fill a box with safe pretzels, cookies, or other treats you allow. Give more than your child needs if possible, to encourage the social benefits of sharing. Next, check in with the classroom parent who organizes special events. Offer to bake an item for class parties if you can, or find out ahead of time what the schedule of these events might be, so you can buy items to share with the class that meet your child's diet restrictions. Like any other parent, make enough for all and share, so your child is just one of the gang on special occasions.

Recipes

This is a not by any stretch a complete collection of recipes, but an odd-ball collection of ideas and items that, over the years, I have fallen upon in obscure places or created myself, and found useful. For soup to nuts suggestions on recipes, a few books are mentioned below, but don't stop there. Almost any recipe can be adjusted to succeed without gluten, casein, soy, or other objectionable ingredients. Look through your own favorite cookbooks and recipes, and experiment with modifying them. Keep on hand an encyclopedic resource such as *The Joy of Cooking* or *Silver Palate Cookbook*. These tell you how to make virtually everything, and then you can cross-reference ingredient substitutions in the books that specialize in the restricted diet genre. Be sure to browse the many websites now up to support users of special diets (some listed earlier in this chapter) for recipes, too.

At Blanchard's Table, by Melinda and Robert Blanchard
Breaking the Vicious Cycle, by Elaine Gottschall
Gluten Free Baking, by Rebecca Reilly
The Gluten-Free Gourmet series of cookbooks, by Bette Hagman
Special Diets for Special Kids, by Lisa Lewis
Stews, from the Williams Sonoma Kitchen Library Collection
The Top One Hundred Pasta Sauces, by Diane Seed
The Victory Garden Cook Book, by Marian Morash

Aside from the obvious dinner ideas that you will easily modify—grilled burgers and hot dogs or bratwurst (with no bun or with gluten-free buns), steaks and fries, spaghetti (gluten-free) and meat sauce, pork roast or pot roast with vegetables (classic, easy, and innately GFCF)—here is a further hodgepodge of recipes. The only criteria for inclusion here is that it worked: it was well liked by just about everybody among my clients, both kids and adults. Some items are here because I found them nowhere else and made them up to fit the diet restrictions. Many parents are gifted in this regard and have done a far better job than I. If you have a flash of brilliance on what's for dinner or a recipe to share, you can post it at www.NutritionCare.net. Most busy families like easy one-dish meals that can feed a family at the end of the day when you haven't figured out what's for dinner, so that is what many of these recipes are about. None of these recipes is new or novel; they simply fit the needs most families may be working with. Besides ideas here, don't forget to build menus out of a main grilled, sautéed, or baked protein (chicken, salmon or other low-mercury fish, pork, beef) and sides such as quinoa or rice salad; grilled, steamed, or broiled vegetables; potato or sweet potato (baked, broiled, fries); and a garden greens salad with your own dressing (which can be fast to make, and can taste better than many bottled versions). Believe it or not, your child may enjoy these "grown-up" foods sooner than you think.

ON FISH AND ORGANIC FOODS. Many families still prefer to allow some fish on their household menus. Whether you choose to still eat fish is a decision for you only. All fish contain some mercury; older, bigger fish have more. Unfortunately, mercury is now ubiquitous in the environment. We are all exposed and retain some. This is not a good thing, and it is a very bad thing for infants and small children, whose developing brains are most vulnerable to this neurotoxin. Mercury exposures you can control are those from medications, foods, dental amalgams, and vaccines. Those you can't control are from coal-burning power plant emissions, industrial pollutants, and agricultural processes and chemicals. For parents who really want a big picture of where mercury is besides vaccines, a report called *Mercury Connections* by the Biodiversity Research Institute in Maine offers an enlightening tally of exactly how pervasive this metal is in our environment. This report details painstakingly measured effects of mercury exposures on fish, birds, and mammals (which showed haunting similarities to features of autism in human children). Mercury may be in many foods besides fish, simply because it is everywhere, and will accumulate in any creature near the top of the food chain.

This is one reason why you might choose organic foods as often as possible. There is no guarantee that mercury is not in those, because no one has yet looked, but assuming the label is honest about a food's organic status, you will be assured of eating fewer chemicals and contaminants. Organic foods usually taste better, too, in my opinion. Ingredients listed in recipes are assumed to be organic, gluten-free, and casein-free.

MINESTRONE IN 20 MINUTES

This recipe is adapted from an offering in Bette Hagman's *Gluten Free Gourmet*, one of a series of cookbooks for persons with celiac disease. Her recipes are easy to modify to accommodate casein restrictions and are, of course, always gluten-free. This version uses fresh herbs and vegetables rather than the original frozen mixed vegetables, and it is still quick to assemble. Vary it more with fresh zuchinni, summer squash, or canned white (cannelli) beans. It is a hearty soup that works well in cold seasons, served with GF rolls or bread. If your crew is really hungry, serve with a grilled bratwurst or favorite GFCF hot dog.

Those who can eat casein can put Parmesan on top when served.

2–3 tablespoons olive oil

2 cloves garlic, or 2 teaspoons minced garlic

2 green onions, chopped

3 tablespoons fresh chopped parsley

1 tablespoon fresh chopped cilantro

5 cups gluten-free beef, chicken, or vegetable broth (Imagine or Pacific brand)

14½-ounce can diced tomatoes

8-ounce can tomato sauce

1 teaspoon dried crushed thyme

¼ teaspoon black pepper

1–2 teaspoons sugar (optional)

1 cup gluten-free pasta (spirals or penne)

2 carrots, chopped

14-ounce can corn, fresh kernels scraped off a cob, or 1 cup frozen

1 cup frozen or fresh green beans

In a large pot, heat oil gently. Sauté garlic, green onions, and fresh herbs until soft. Add broth, tomatoes, tomato sauce, thyme, pepper, and sugar (if used). Bring to a boil. Add the remaining ingredients. Simmer uncovered until the pasta is cooked, about 15 minutes. Serve with Chébé rolls or breadsticks, or Kinnikinnick pizza rounds prepared as focaccia. (Bake these from your freezer for 12 minutes at 350 degrees after spraying or brushing with olive oil and seasoning with basil, oregano, garlic powder, salt, and black pepper.)

PORTUGUESE KALE SOUP

Kale is a great source of vitamin K. Make a big batch of this soup so that it has a couple days to really set its flavors. This recipe is virtually public domain and the one below is an amalgam from several sources plus what works in my kitchen. Use a food processor to get through the onion chopping without tears, if you like.

> 5 larger red potatoes or 4 big baker potatoes
> 1 pound sliced chourico (aka chorizo, Portuguese sausage, or linguica)
> ¼ cup olive oil
> 2 large yellow onions, chopped
> 6 cloves garlic, crushed, or 2 tablespoons minced garlic
> 1 bay leaf
> 1 pound kale
> 1 can red kidney beans
> 6 cups chicken broth
> salt and pepper to taste
> 28-ounce can chopped tomatoes (optional)

Peel and chop the potatoes into half-inch cubes. Parboil them (boil about 5 minutes) in enough water to cover them. In a separate pan, sauté the sliced chourico in the olive oil. Add the onion, garlic, and bay leaf; do not let the garlic burn or brown. Add the sautéed ingredients to the potatoes and the water they were boiled in, turning the heat down to simmer. Add the remaining ingredients except the tomatoes. Let simmer for 10 minutes, then add the tomatoes. Continue cook on low simmer for about an hour. Serve with gluten-free bread in a big bowl for a meal in itself, or as a side with a light, low-mercury fish such as baked or broiled cod or a few scallops.

Meat Loaf

Adapted from Yankee Magazine's
Favorite New England Recipes (Second Edition)

What can I say? It's good. This ultimate-in-the-pedestrian entrée is always appreciated when it's done right. The texture is melt-in-your-mouth and savory. Serve with quinoa cooked in chicken broth with minced santéed mushrooms added, and a garden salad. Or try serving with herbed and broiled new potatoes, mashed potatoes made GFCF, or steamed patty pan squash. The cookbook from which I've pulled this reliable recipe is intriguing. In it there are instructions for everything from how to make a Christmas Bag Pudding ("really give it a larruping") to a recipe for Lobster Coral Sauce (which requires the female's roe and cognac). If you enjoy obscure recipes and a historical perspective on American cooking, see if you can dig this book up.

> 1 pound ground beef
> 2–3 slices gluten-free sandwich bread, spun to fine texture in a food processor
> 1 onion, minced (chopped fine or in a food processor)
> 2 tablespoons fresh parsley, minced
> 1 clove fresh minced or 1 teaspoon minced garlic
> 2 eggs
> 1 cup tomato sauce or gluten-free tomato soup
> 1½ teaspoons salt
> fresh ground black pepper
> tomato catsup
> 3 strips gluten-free bacon

Mix all ingredients together until well blended, except the catsup and the bacon. Press into a greased bread loaf ban. Spread a thin layer of catsup over the surface of the loaf. You can also bake this as a loaf on a cookie sheet. Arrange bacon strips on the surface of the loaf. Bake at 375 degrees for 45 minutes.

Pork Long Bean

This is an adaptation of a staple Chinese menu item. True afficionados of this dish will have their own approach; check online for other versions and experiment. Long bean is available in Asian markets. Each bean is like a green whip, a foot long or longer. Buy them thinner and shorter so they will be more tender. If they are over 18 inches long, they may be tough (they are still good if you cook them longer). Pork is a good source of protein and minerals, while the long bean also offers some protein, B vitamins, potassium, iron, folate, magnesium, and manganese.

1 bunch long bean (about ¾ pound)
1 pound 90 percent lean ground pork
2 cloves garlic, or 2 teaspoons minced garlic
1 small onion, quartered
3 slices fresh ginger
½ teaspoon red curry paste (Thai Kitchen brand)
1 tablespoon wheat-free tamari
salt and pepper to taste
coconut milk (optional)

Wash the long bean and cut into four-inch segments. If they are thicker and longer beans, cook partway through in a pot with a vegetable steamer, or covered with some water in a microwave. If they are younger, smaller, and tender, you do not need to precook. Simmer the pork with garlic, onion, ginger, and curry paste until some fat is rendered out of it, about 5 minutes. Add the tamari. If it needs it, salt to taste, and do not overcook. Grind fresh black pepper into the mix and add the long bean. Cook until the long bean is tender and slightly crisp. Add more tamari if you like. Serve with sticky rice.

OPTION: You may add a can of unsweetened coconut milk to the pork at the beginning of the recipe.

CORN CHOWDER

Adapted from At Blanchard's Table

This is easy, light, and fast. It is not the cream-reliant version you may be expecting.

3 tablespoons ghee, olive oil, or Earth Balance margarine

3 medium yellow onions, chopped

5 carrots, cut into ¼-inch slices

5 celery stalks, cut into ¼-inch slices

6 cups fresh corn kernels off the cob (canned or frozen are okay, too)

1 quart chicken broth (Imagine or Pacific brand)

¾ teaspoon salt

½ teaspoon fresh ground black pepper

2 large red bell peppers, seeded and cut into ½-inch slivers

3 tablespoons chopped fresh dill

Heat the ghee, oil, or margarine in a large pot. When hot, add the onions, carrots, and celery and cook until tender (you may precook the carrots in a microwave, steaming them with a little hot water, to speed this up). Sauté about 10 minutes then add the corn to cook 2 minutes more. Remove about two-thirds of the vegetables, and transfer to a food processor. Puree until smooth and return to the pot. Add the broth, salt, and pepper, and bring to a boil. As soon as it boils, add the red peppers and dill and simmer for 2 more minutes. Serve hot, with gluten-free bread. Good along with grilled chicken or Chicken Picatta.

CHICKEN PICATTA

This was given to me by a friend, photocopied from a magazine years ago. We adapted it to be GFCF and to include more calories from fats and oils. Serves six. Good with fresh steamed green beans or snap peas, broiled zucchini, garden salad, and rice or risotto. Feels heartier when paired with baked sweet potatoes.

gluten-free flour blend of 2 parts brown rice flour, 1/2 part tapioca starch, and 1/2 part potato flour; about 1/2 to 2/3 cup

salt and fresh ground pepper

pinch of corn meal

1 1/2 pounds boneless chicken breasts or tenders

1 tablespoon olive oil and 1 tablespoon ghee

1/4 cup dry white wine

2 cloves garlic, or 2 teaspoons minced garlic

1/2 cup gluten-free chicken broth (Imagine or Pacific brand)

2 tablespoons lemon juice

1 tablespoon capers, drained (optional)

fresh lemon slices

Make enough gluten-free flour blend for dusting all the chicken, about 1/2 cup. Mix into the flour blend several grinds of black pepper, salt, and the corn meal. Dust the cutlets well. Heat the oil or fat in a large, deep skillet to medium high. Sauté the chicken in the skillet for about 2 minutes on each side. Do not cook through. Transfer cutlets to a warm plate and cover with a pot lid or kitchen towel. Deglaze the skillet with the wine and add the garlic. Cook until garlic is just beginning to brown (don't burn or brown), about 2 minutes. Add chicken broth, lemon juice, and capers if you are using them. Return cutlets to the skillet. Place fresh lemon slices atop the chicken and continue at low simmer until chicken is cooked, about 5 minutes. Chicken should be very tender.

GARBANZO PASTA CURRY

This is a fast, easy dinner that will be enjoyed once children accept mixed foods. Serve with gluten-free bread and a small bowl of Imagine or Pacific brand ready-to-heat butternut squash soup for a fuller meal.

 2 tablespoons olive oil
 1 onion, chopped
 2 cloves garlic, or 2 teaspoons minced garlic
 1 green bell pepper, chopped
 2 teaspoons chili powder
 1 teaspoon curry powder
 ½ pound lean ground beef (grass-fed organic if you can get it)
 28-ounce can chopped tomatoes
 1 cup gluten-free tomato or meatless spaghetti sauce
 16-ounce can garbanzo beans (chickpeas)
 3 cups gluten-free pasta (corkscrew)
 salt and fresh ground pepper

Heat the olive oil in a deep skillet. Add the onion, garlic, pepper, chili powder, and curry powder. Sauté until the onion is clear. Add the ground beef and cook until some fat is rendered. Add tomatoes, tomato sauce, and beans. Let simmer on low heat. Meanwhile, cook the pasta. Drain and mix with garbanzo curry. Serve hot.

BASIL CHICKEN SPAGHETTI

Adapted from The Top One Hundred Pasta Sauces

Before anyone realized eating a lot of tuna was probably a bad idea (owing to mercury content), this recipe was pressed into service often in our house—another easy, fast dinner. The original recipe called for a can of tuna, which sounds worse than meat loaf. But with lemon rind and fresh herbs, it works well. Now we use chicken in place of tuna and use more basil than in the original recipe.

> 7-ounce can white chicken meat, or same amount of cooked chopped chicken
>
> ½ cup walnuts if tolerated; try pine nuts if not
>
> grated rind of 1 lemon
>
> 1 teaspoon Worcestershire sauce
>
> 2 tablespoons fresh chopped parsley
>
> 2 tablespoons fresh chopped basil leaves
>
> ¾ cup (6 ounces) high-quality olive oil
>
> salt and black pepper
>
> gluten-free spaghetti for four

Put drained chicken meat, nuts, lemon rind, Worcestershire, and herbs into a food processor or blender and process until smooth. Add the olive oil gradually, and adjust seasoning with salt and pepper to taste. Stir into the just-cooked hot pasta and coat each strand of spaghetti. Also good on penne pasta, and served with a vibrant mixed greens salad.

SPRING ROLLS

These are labor-intensive but worth it when you have time and don't mind making a pretty good mess in your kitchen. Kids love them. Once you have the sequence of the recipe down, it's not difficult. A food processor makes this easier.

½ cup cooked ham, ground pork, or chicken, finely minced in a food processor

½ small package of bean thread, soaked and chopped

2 scallions (green onions), chopped

4-ounce can of water chestnuts, minced

2 tablespoons bean or lentil sprouts

1 stalk celery, minced

½ teaspoon minced garlic

2 tablespoons gluten-free soy sauce (tamari)

salt and pepper

12–15 small spring roll skins (Red Rose brand— "Banh Trang")

water

1 egg, beaten

safflower oil

Mix all but the last four ingredients, chopped and minced, together in a bowl with tamari, salt, and pepper. Set aside. In a large pot, pour water to 1-inch depth and heat until it's hot to the touch. One at a time, soak spring roll skins in the warm water until just soft, 10–30 seconds. Remove each skin from the water and lay it on a cutting board or other flat surface. Add 2 tablespoons of minced ingredients as filling. Roll the spring roll skin, like a burrito, two-thirds of the way, then fold the ends in around the filling. Finish rolling by using your fingertip to brush beaten egg on the remaining edge. Then close up the egg roll by pressing the remaining edge onto the roll.

Pour oil to ¾-inch depth in a large, deep pot over medium-high heat. When drops of water spatter in the oil, it is hot enough. Fry the spring rolls in the oil until lightly browned and crispy, 1–2 minutes per side. Drain on paper towels and serve with steamed rice. A deep fryer may be used instead of a deep pot if you own one.

RATATOUILLE

Adapted from The Victory Garden Cook Book

A satisfying old standby that is filling in itself, but especially when served with whole grain brown rice or gluten-free bread. Grilled apple chicken sausage rounds this out as a meal. Ratatouille will really sing when the ingredients are at their best. If you have access to fresh local vegetables at the peak of ripeness, try this recipe. This version adds herbs. *The Victory Garden Cook Book* is great for illustrating how to incorporate more vegetables into main dishes and meals.

1 pound eggplant
1 pound zucchini
salt
1 pound onions
¼ pound green and red bell peppers
1 pound ripe tomatoes
⅓ cup good-quality olive oil
1 tablespoon minced garlic
fresh ground pepper
½ teaspoon dried oregano (try fresh minced oregano, too, if you have it)
½ teaspoon dried basil (a few big fresh leaves, slivered, are also good)

Peel the eggplant and cut into ½-inch cubes. Wash the zucchini and do the same. Toss both with salt and let drain for 30 minutes. Meanwhile, slice the onions; clean the peppers and sliver, or chop into ½-inch pieces. Chop the tomatoes into quarters (you can peel and seed them before chopping if you prefer). Dry the eggplant and zucchini by pressing out the remaining water with a paper towel.

Heat about half the oil in a large sauté pan. Add the eggplant and brown on all sides. Add the zucchini and peppers and sauté for 5 minutes. Remove the vegetables from the pan into a big bowl and set aside. Add the remaining oil and sauté the onions until they are wilted. Stir in garlic and tomatoes, and cover the pan. Cook for 4 minutes, uncover the pan, and raise the heat until juices evaporate. Season generously with salt, pepper, and spices, then add back vegetables that were set aside. Cover and simmer for 10–15 minutes and baste occasionally. Serve hot. Leftover ratatouille is good on pizza rounds or spooned into omelettes.

CHICKEN TERIYAKI

A basic. Serve with any favorite sides. If you can find black rice, try it, or mix it with steamed white rice. Black rice turns a purplish black when cooked, has a fragrant nutty flavor, and has a better amino acid profile than white rice. It also contains iron.

¼ cup gluten-free soy sauce (tamari)
½ cup olive oil
1 teaspoon honey
1 teaspoon brown sugar
1 teaspoon minced garlic
4–6 thin slices fresh ginger root
1 ½ cups warm water
1 pound boneless chicken tenders

Mix all ingredients, except chicken, in a glass bowl. Mix until sugar and honey are dissolved and evenly dispersed. Place chicken tenders in marinade and immerse them as much as possible. Cover tightly with plastic wrap and let sit at room temperature for 30 minutes, or you may refrigerate for up to 6–8 hours. When ready to cook, place on a hot grill or under a broiler for 2 minutes per side. Makes 2 large or 3 small servings.

MILD CURRY CHICKEN

Another easy way to use coconut milk. The mild and sweet curry is usually a hit with kids.

 1 onion, chopped fine
 1/2 cup chopped celery
 1/2 cup chopped carrots
 1/2 cup chopped sweet red or green pepper
 2 tablespoons olive oil or clarified butter (ghee)
 1 quart gluten-free chicken broth (Imagine or Pacific brand)
 1 cup water
 2 large bay leaves
 1/2 teaspoon curry powder
 1/2 teaspoon dried thyme
 1/4 teaspoon allspice
 1/8 teaspoon ground black pepper
 1/2 cup Minute Rice
 1 pound boneless skinless chicken, cubed
 1 can unsweetened coconut milk
 1 can black beans
 2 tablespoons sugar (optional)

In a large pot, sauté the onion, celery, carrots, and peppers in the ghee/oil. Add the broth, water, bay leaves, and spices. Bring to a boil. Add the rice; cover and simmer for 10 minutes. Add the cubed chicken to the pot and simmer for 5 minutes. Add the coconut milk, canned beans, and optional sugar. Simmer through and serve.

TACOS WITH LIME CHICKEN

You don't need cheese to make good tacos. Guacamole, avocado slices, and black olive slices lend a similar texture and satiety. Use soft corn tortillas for kids who don't like crunchy. They can roll up their own at the table if that is engaging and fun. Serve with steamed rice and cooked corn.

2 tablespoons olive oil

2 teaspoons garlic

1 pound leftover teriyaki chicken, roast chicken, or baked chicken

2 tablespoons lime juice

pinch sugar (optional)

¼ cup chopped fresh cilantro

chopped fresh tomato

chopped fresh lettuce

1 cup guacamole or 1 ripe avocado

1 can refried beans

1 small can black olive slices

tomato salsa (your preference, mild to hot)

8 corn taco shells

Heat the olive oil in a skillet. Add the garlic and heat gently; do not brown. Finely chop the chicken and add to the skillet. Heat through. Add the lime juice, sugar, and 1 tablespoon of the chopped cilantro. Cover and allow to gently heat through. Meanwhile, chop the tomato and lettuce, and set these plus guacamole/sliced avocado, refried beans, olives, remaining cilantro, and salsa on your table in any way you'd like so everyone can build his or her own tacos—on one large platter, in separate dishes, or a combination. Bake the taco shells in a 350-degree oven for 4 minutes. Place on the table with chicken filling. Refried beans are good either in the tacos or on the side.

BROILED ZUCCHINI

Wash fresh zucchini and cut it lengthwise into halves or thirds. Spray or brush with good olive oil, then dust with garlic salt, dried oregano, and dried basil. Place under 400-degree broiler until browned, about 8 minutes.

BAKED SWEET POTATO

Just as you would prepare an Idaho baker, bake these for a variation on the usual side dish. Children often like the sweeter flavor. Wash fresh sweet potatoes, and cut into large pieces (halves) or leave whole. Bake in a 400-degree oven until done, about an hour. You can also partly cook these in the microwave first, then finish with baking, if you are in a hurry. Don't overlook sweet potato fries, now available in the frozen food section of most supermarkets, as a welcome (and healthful) variation on the old favorite.

RICE, QUINOA, OR GLUTEN-FREE PASTA SALADS

Mix any ingredients your family may like and use rice as the vehicle for a side dish. Experiment with different dressings, or serving warm or chilled. This is my current favorite. Other ingredients to consider are black beans, green beans, sesame seeds, heirloom tomatoes, or other fresh herbs. This recipe has traveled successfully to winter potlucks and summer picnics, and the bowl usually comes home empty.

> 6 cups cooked sticky rice
> 2 green onions, chopped
> 1/4 cup chopped fresh cilantro
> 12 cherry or grape tomatoes, halved
> 1 can wax beans or 1 1/2 cups fresh steamed wax beans
> 1 cup green peas, lightly steamed (still with a crunch)
> 2 tablespoons minced black olives
> 2 teaspoons minced garlic
> 1 can coconut milk
> 1/2 cup Brianna's Honey Mustard bottled dressing
> salt and fresh ground pepper to taste

When rice is cooked and warm, mix all ingredients together in a big bowl. Combine thoroughly so everything is covered by the coconut milk and the dressing.

BAKED HERBED NEW POTATOES

Another way to round out a main protein. Many kids like these reheated under the broiler or in a skillet at breakfast.

    12 new potatoes (the smaller red ones!)
    1 green bell pepper
    1 large onion
    garlic or garlic salt
    fresh ground black pepper
    fresh chopped dill or dried dill spice
    1/2 cup olive oil

Chop the potatoes into bite-size pieces. Put in a microwave-safe bowl and cook on high for 5 minutes or until partly cooked. Meanwhile, chop the onion and green pepper but not too fine. When the potatoes come out of the microwave, combine in a large bowl with the remaining ingredients. Mix thoroughly to coat everything with oil and spices. Bake in a 400-degree oven for 20–25 minutes.

Vegetable Tempura

Adapted from Bette Hagman's
More from the Gluten Free Gourmet

You might get some picky eaters on board by presenting vegetables as tempura. This brings out the natural sweetness in carrots, onions, asparagus, broccoli bits, and fresh green beans. For carrots, shred or cut them julienne, dip clumps in batter with a slotted spoon, and lower into hot oil. The soda in this recipe imparts necessary crispness and browning, thanks to its sugar content and carbonation. Allow it now and then and don't sweat it. If you'd like to stay really natural with this part, try Jones soda, which uses cane sugar and not corn syrup. To avoid the sugar, try their sugar-free version, which uses Sucralose and not aspartame (a neurotoxin) as a sweetener.

1 egg, beaten
¼ cup cornstarch
½ cup sweet rice flour
¼ teaspoon xanthan gum
1 teaspoon salt
½ teaspoon baking powder
1 cup ginger ale or Sprite
3 cups vegetable oil for deep frying
2–3 cups washed cut vegetables

In a medium bowl, beat the egg. Mix the cornstarch, rice flour, xanthan gum, salt, and baking powder. Stir the dry mix into the egg alternately with the ginger ale or Sprite. Heat the oil in a frying pan until it is 375 degrees. Dip the vegetables in batter, then gently drop into the hot oil. Cook 3–5 minutes, turning once as they brown. Allow longer cooking if necessary. Remove and drain on a paper towel. Serve hot, and add a dipping sauce if you like.

Instant Sides of Yams

Empty one or two cans of yams into a pot. Heat while mashing with a potato masher. The syrup these are packed in can be used to sweeten and soften the yams, for kids who will accept only smooth, sweet textures. You can also rinse and drain the yams and add back a sweetener of your choice such as a bit of honey or maple syrup.

Beets

Beets are a naturally sweet carbohydrate that are easy to present to children directly out of the can and plated, julienned and added to garden salads, or even roasted. Fresh sliced from the garden, like most vegetables, they offer flavor that explains why people used to eat a lot more vegetables than they do now. If you have a pressure cooker, you can steam fresh sliced beets in about 10 minutes. They have a soft, uniform texture that is easy for children who can't tolerate variations in that regard. Try this version, from *At Blanchard's Table*:

8 small fresh beets
1 1/2 tablespoons gluten-free apple cider vinegar
3 tablespoons olive oil
1/2 teaspoon gluten-free Dijon mustard
1/2 cup whole cranberry sauce
salt and pepper
goat cheese crumbles (if tolerated)

Preheat oven to 400 degrees. Cut off beet greens, leaving an inch of stem. Wrap each beet individually in foil. Roast them on a baking sheet until tender, 60–90 minutes; they will feel soft when squeezed lightly. Unwrap and cool to room temperature. Peel and cut into quarter-inch-thick slices. In a small bowl, whisk together remaining ingredients. Toss the beets with the dressing and mound on a plate. Those who can tolerate goat cheese might crumble some on top. Serve at room temperature.

Sauces and Dressings

Making your own can become a habit. They are not so time-consuming after all. You control the ingredients, and they often taste better. Here are a few.

Creamy Lime Dressing

from The New Basics Cookbook

This is handy for both fruit and green garden salads, and as a vegetable dip for kids previously hooked on ranch (dairy) dressings. Makes 2½ cups. Halve the recipe to have plenty of dressing for one garden salad that serves 4–6 people.

> 5 tablespoons lime juice
> 2 eggs
> 2 tablespoons gluten-free Dijon mustard
> 1 cup good olive oil
> 1 cup safflower oil
> grated zest of 2 limes
> fresh ground black pepper
> pinch of sugar (optional)

Place lime juice, eggs, and mustard in a food processor and process for 15 seconds. With the motor running, slowly add the oils and process until thickened; it will take on the consistency of mayonnaise or aioli. Transfer to a bowl and fold in the lime zest, pepper, and optional sugar.

GINGER TAHINI DRESSING

Good on a simple garden salad with mixed bold greens, dried orange essence cranberries, scallions, and julienned cucumber. Also a good dip for fresh green, red, or yellow peppers, and cucumbers, too—two vegetables that children seem to open up to early on in the nutrition care game, for their juicy crunch and mild sweetness.

  ½ cup good olive oil
  3–4 slices fresh ginger
  ½ teaspoon minced garlic
  1–2 teaspoons gluten-free balsamic vinegar
  1 tablespoon orange juice
  2 tablespoons tahini
  2 tablespoons Brianna's Honey Mustard bottled dressing
  pinch of sugar (optional)

Pour the olive oil into a small pitcher, dressing bottle, or cup with hand blender. Add ginger and garlic. Add vinegar and whisk briefly. Add remaining ingredients and whisk or blend until smooth.

MILD RED THAI CURRY SAUCE

Adapted from At Blanchard's Table

This recipe is presented in the Blanchards' book as an accompaniment to grilled mahi, which you can now buy at Costco vacuum-packed and frozen. If you're skipping that, it is also good with grilled chicken. The original calls for peanut oil, which I've replaced here since so many kids are sensitized to it, and more heat, which I've toned down for kids also.

3 tablespoons olive or safflower oil

1/2 teaspoon sesame oil

1 clove garlic

1 1/2 teaspoons fresh ginger, peeled and minced

2 teaspoons curry powder

2 teaspoons Thai red curry paste (Thai Kitchen brand is gluten-free and in most supermarkets)

1/2 teaspoon paprika

1/2 teaspoon ground cumin

2 tablespoons gulten-free soy sauce (tamari)

2 tablespoons tomato puree

2 tablespoons packed light brown sugar

1 can unsweetened coconut milk

Have all your ingredients measured and ready at the stove. In a large saucepan, heat the oils over medium heat. Add the garlic and ginger, and cook for 1 minute. Reduce heat to low, and add the curry powder, paste, paprika, and cumin. Stir and cook for 2 minutes. Raise the heat back to medium and add the tamari, tomato puree, brown sugar, and coconut milk, whisking well at each addition. When small bubbles form around the edge of the pan, simmer on low heat for 10 minutes, whisking frequently. Do not boil. Brush the sauce on fish or chicken and grill. Serve with extra sauce over rice and a side of corn and fresh mango slices, if you can get them.

DIPS

Kids who like only crunchy chips can sometimes be transitioned to better choices when a compelling dip is offered. Move from dairy-based ranch salad dressings to the Creamy Lime version given in this chapter, then on to new flavors. Hummus and other bean dips are great for calories and protein, and you can add extra olive oil and lemon juice to further enhance flavor and calories. Offer with bell pepper slices, carrot, celery, corn chips, raw young asparagus, or rice crackers. Here is a recipe from *At Blanchard's Table* that incorporates bacon.

WHITE BEAN DIP

1 can cannellini beans

1–2 teaspoons lemon juice

1 teaspoon water, if needed

4 strips cooked bacon (gluten- and nitrite/nitrate-free)

1 tablespoon minced black olives (available ready to use in small cans)

fresh or dried thyme

salt and pepper

Blend the beans in a food processor with 1 teaspoon of the lemon juice. Add more lemon juice to taste, and additional water if you need it, to make a creamy smooth mixture. Crumble or mince the bacon. Transfer the bean mixture to a bowl and stir in the bacon, olives, and sprinkling of dried thyme. Add salt and pepper to taste. Garnish with a few dots of fresh thyme and some parsley if you have it. Try dipping baby carrots, fresh bell pepper slices, cucumbers cut in sticks or coins, celery, or gluten-free items like taco chips, rice crackers, Blue Diamond Nut Thins, or Glutino Mini Bread Sticks.

DESSERTS AND TREATS

Nobody's perfect, least of all kids with special diet needs. Kids need breaks, indulgences, treats, and participation in the foods of special occasions. Allow transgressions for sweets within reason. Unless your child endangers his safety with a treat—as a diabetic might do when eating a sweet without appropriate coverage from an insulin dose— you may do your child more harm than good if you are relentlessly rigid on this part. As mentioned earlier, mixes and recipes abound for baked goods that are gluten-free, and casein substitutes in those recipes are straightforward. Here are several ideas that stand out for a special day.

MOLTEN CHOCOLATE CAKES

Adapted from Gluten Free Baking

The consensus so far, among neighbors, clients, family, and school classmates is that these are really good and in no way inferior to a version that uses wheat flour. Rebecca Reilly's recipe in *Gluten Free Baking* is called Warm Chocolate Hazelnut Cake. Since a hazelnut sensitivity is an issue for some, try this substitute approach with almond flour, but either works. Among tree nuts, almonds are less likely to be allergenic. Serve with fresh raspberries or a raspberry fruit puree for a nice finish.

> 4 ounces casein-free bittersweet chocolate
> 1 ounce unsweetened baker's chocolate
> 1 stick (½ cup) casein-free margarine or ghee
> 2 eggs
> 2 egg yolks
> ¼ cup sugar
> 1 tablespoon almond flour or hazelnut flour

Preheat oven to 450 degrees. Lightly coat individual brioche tins (if you have them) or a muffin tray for six large muffins (if you don't) with cooking spray. Melt the chocolates and margarine together. Beat the eggs, egg yolks, and sugar until they are thick and pale yellow, and form about a half-inch-wide ribbon when you lift the beater—this will take a few minutes! Beat in the warm melted chocolate and butter mixture. Quickly fold in the flour you are using. Spoon into prepared molds. Bake 6–7 minutes. The centers will be soft, the sides firm. Invert onto a flat surface (directly onto dessert plates if you have those brioche tins; or onto a smooth cutting board if you don't) and let cool for about 10 minutes before unmolding. Serve with fruit if you like.

PUMPKIN BREAD

This is also adapted from *Gluten Free Baking*, with the only changes made here to accommodate the casein restriction. Makes an easy calorie-dense snack for children, with the benefit of ingredients such as pumpkin and nuts, for those who can have them.

1¾ cups gluten-free flour mix for baking
(2 parts brown rice flour, ⅔ part potato starch,
⅓ part tapioca starch)

1 teaspoon baking soda

1 teaspoon xanthan gum

½ teaspoon cinnamon

¼ teaspoon gluten-free baking powder

¼ teaspoon cloves

⅛ teaspoon nutmeg

pinch powdered ginger

⅓ cup casein-free margarine or ghee

1⅓ cups packed light brown sugar

2 eggs

1 cup pumpkin puree (canned is fine)

⅓ cup almond, hazelnut, or vanilla soy milk

½ cup chopped macadamia nuts (or other nuts, raisins,
dates, or cranberries as you prefer)

Preheat oven to 350 degrees. Lightly grease a 9 × 5-inch loaf pan and dust it with rice flour, or line it with baking parchment. You can also use a muffin tin; line 12 muffin cups with paper liners. Mix together the GF flour mix, baking soda, xanthan gum, cinnamon, baking powder, cloves, nutmeg, and ginger. Cream the margarine until white. Add the sugar and beat until fluffy (about 5 minutes). Add the eggs, one at a time. If the mixture appears cracked, add 1 or 2 tablespoons of the dry ingredients until it looks smooth. Stir in the pumpkin puree. Add the dry ingredients, alternating with the milk substitute. Add chopped nuts or fruit. Spoon the batter into the prepared loaf pan or muffin tins. Bake the loaf for 1 hour, small loaves for 25 minutes, or muffins 15–18 minutes.

FLAKY PASTRY PIECRUST

From *Gluten Free Baking*

I made several attempts at gluten-free piecrusts over the years, which guests graciously ate, until finding Rebecca Reilly's book and using her recipe below. Rebecca Reilly is a trained chef and pastry maker who found herself needing to accommodate gluten intolerance in her children; thus her book was born. The butter is adapted to be casein-free. This is a case where you may do well to splurge on the ghee (clarified butter), as casein-free margarine will be too soft. Use this crust for holiday fruit pies, pumpkin pies, mince pies, or quiches that are allowable for those who avoid gluten but not dairy. Makes a single crust. For piecrusts, I like the bite of the bean flours, so I use that in my flour mix by blending it as follows: 1½ cups brown rice flour, ½ cup bean flour, ⅔ cup potato starch, and ⅓ tapioca starch. From this I pull the 1 cup of gluten-free flour blend used in the recipe.

1 cup basic gluten-free flour mix

2 tablespoons sweet rice flour

1½ teaspoons sugar

¼ teaspoon salt

6 tablespoons cold unsalted ghee

1 egg

1 tablespoon cider vinegar or lemon juice

Mix together the gluten-free flour mix, sweet rice flour, sugar, and salt. Cut the ghee into chunks, and using your fingertips, work it into the dry ingredients to form a coarse meal. Make a well. Break the egg into the well. Add the vinegar or lemon juice. Use a fork to stir from the center, working the flour into the egg to form a soft dough. Shape into a flat cake. Cover and chill in the refrigerator for an hour or so, if too soft to roll out. When it is ready, dust a flat surface with gluten-free flour or rice flour, and roll it out. I have had more success getting the rolled crust into a pie plate by spreading a sheet of wax paper on my kitchen island, fixing the corners so it won't move, and dusting it as a surface for rolling. I also frequently dust the roller itself if needed. When the crust is about a quarter-inch thick, I invert the wax paper so I can lay the crust on the greased pie plate in one piece. The wax paper should then easily peel off, allowing you to lightly press the crust into the dish, and to crimp or flute the edges of the crust as you like.

INFANT FORMULA

Infant formula is a tightly controlled and regulated food, as it should be. Babies should not be given substitutes for breast milk that are not suited to their unique per-pound needs for correct levels and types of protein, fat, carbohydrate, vitamins, and minerals. Milks from rice, hemp, soy, oat, or nuts are not safe or suitable for infants. Unfortunately, as a new mom, I found myself in a situation where I had to actually create a formula for my son. I was not wanting to do this but was simply left with no options. Though Neocate (elemental amino acid–based) formula may have helped him, no one offered it and I didn't know about it in 1996. Semi-elemental formula (such as Nutramigen) was successful only for a short while, then it, too, triggered problems. Soy also seemed fine at first, only to become another misfire. On it, my five-month-old son simply stopped eliminating any stool. He endured twelve days of passing no bowel movements at all, after passing fewer and fewer dry, small hard stools after perhaps three weeks on soy formula. He passed a dusty, dry, stone-like stool before making none at all for days, and nearly stopped eating entirely. He was clearly in pain and distressed; his appetite dwindled more each day, as his belly bloated harder and bigger; and his eczema returned with it, too. I was dumbfounded that my pediatrician had nothing to offer me when I called for further instruction. When I asked for another strategy, he told me "not to worry, the soy formula is fine" and that this was "just a comfort issue."

This triggered one of the biggest epiphanies for me as a parent, and a nutritionist. How could a doctor who is responsible for the well-being of infants and children say such a thing? A baby who cannot eat enough or eliminate any stool for twelve days is not fine, and it astounded me that a doctor would think otherwise. I hung up on him, and resolved to find an answer myself. We'd made it to six months on breast milk, but my son needed a food that would permit him to recover good growth and developmental tasking, both of which were limping along at reduced expectations. In 1996, there was no goat milk infant formula information a second or two away via the Internet, but goat milk still became my choice to work with for creating a formula. After old-fashioned, painstaking research on its nutrient content and benefits, I created a formula that matched human milk for calories per ounce and ratios of macronutrients. To this day, there is no commercial goat milk infant formula available, but a few recipes are on the Web, including a version that is virtually the same as the one I created years ago. You can try any one of them, and unlike me years ago, you can probably have your provider's input and support.

Like cow's milk, straight-up goat's milk can't be given to infants under one year, but it can be incorporated into a recipe that is gentle enough and nutritious for babies. The casein in it is more similar to human milk casein than cow casein, and is thus much easier on the baby's stomach; the fat in it is easier to digest and absorb than cow's milk fat. It was the charm my son needed. He began smiling, chirping, and chubbed up for the first time. He was free to sleep a bit better and look around, too, rather than withdraw as he had been doing, into pain, exhaustion, irritability, or anxiety. He was only six months old, but we were delighted to see him feeling better and happier, and engaging more with his surroundings and his family.

I have added improvements to this recipe that I didn't know about back then, such as probiotics and better choices for oils and carbohydrate sources. Vitamin drops are necessary, as goat milk is slight for key nutrients such as folic acid and vitamin B12. If your infant or young toddler has not been able to tolerate breast milk or commercial formulas, this is an option worth considering. Tell your licensed health care provider about it before you begin and get her input first. If she is unfamiliar with this approach, share the nutrition information included here, to reassure her that this is a safe substitute for breast milk, in terms of calories, protein, fats, carbohydrate, and levels for vitamins and minerals.

GOAT MILK INFANT FORMULA

This recipe makes 8 ounces of goat milk infant formula, which provides approximately 170 calories, 5 grams of protein, 9 grams of fat, and 10–11 grams of carbohydrate. This is nearly identical to the macronutrient profile of human milk. Flax oil adds valuable DHA, and probiotic powder aids your baby's digestion. Review the suggestions for vitamin and mineral additions below with your pediatrician.

> 5 ounces reconstituted powdered goat milk (Meyenberg brand)
>
> 3 ounces water
>
> 1 teaspoon flax oil
>
> 1 teaspoon sunflower or safflower oil
>
> 1/2 tablespoon Lundberg brand Brown Rice Syrup
>
> 1/8 teaspoon *Bifidobacterium infantis* (probiotic)

Once daily, add a dose of infant vitamin drops, such as Twin Labs Infant Care Multi with DHÅ. Allow up to a half teaspoon total probiotic daily, but start with a low dose. Going too fast with a probiotic can cause diarrhea. Goat milk is low in folic acid, so you will want to add this as well; it is not in infant vitamin drops as it is assumed present in breast milk or formula. You can purchase a trial size of Kirkman Labs Liquid Folinic Acid with Methy-B12, and give a few drops or up to a quarter teaspoon daily. Babies normally do not need iron supplements, as they are born with stored iron obtained from Mom. If you suspect you had poor iron status during pregnancy, review with your doctor whether or not your baby should receive iron. Iron is toxic in the wrong dose, so do not add this to formula without medical supervision. Infant vitamins do not typically provide minerals. Occasionally adding a few drops of tasteless liquid zinc (Metagenics brand Zinc Drink) can be helpful. When your baby reaches the one-year mark, it is a good time to review her growth and feeding, and discuss what changes might be needed. It is common for parents not to give enough solids at this age but to continue offering a lot of fluid calories, simply out of habit—but young toddlers need more solid calories than they did even a couple months earlier.

Smoothies for Kids with Diet Restrictions

Smoothies you make at home can be a good way to pack in nutrients your child won't eat. You can add flax oil, probiotic powder, amino acid powder or protein powder, or supplements, as long as the flavor does not become objectionable. Some parents even add fish oil supplements to smoothies or juices. Fruit sorbets have sugar, of course, but can help your child accept some other important calories or micronutrients, and provide a thick base for you to work with. A convenient way to do this is to use a frozen whole fruit bar: Microwave it upside down in a large glass for a few seconds to soften it, then pull out the wooden stick, and add your other ingredients to make the smoothie (juice, coconut milk, etc.) and blend with a hand blender. Kirkman Labs sells GFCF flavorings that use Sucralose as the sweetener, for kids who need to control sugars. You can also experiment with unsweetened coconut milk, sesame tahini, peanut butter, or other tolerated nut butters for smoothies, or add boosts like Ultracare for Kids from Metagenics. Fresh fruit or juice-packed canned fruit blended in a smoothie works well, too. I have added eggs to smoothies also, because they provide high-quality protein and fat, and impart body and creaminess, just as they do in salad dressings (as in the Creamy Lime recipe I've given in this chapter). I'm not supposed to tell anyone to eat raw eggs. The FDA notes that one in twenty thousand eggs may contain bad bacteria. It is thus perhaps easier to encounter rotten cream, milk, or contaminated tomatoes than bad eggs. You can check eggs for freshness by lowering them gently into water. If they float, do not use them. If they sink, bacteria are not fermenting inside. Older eggs also have more watery, thinning whites; fresher eggs have whites that stand up with a more gel-like appearance. If you use raw eggs, buy the freshest, highest-quality local organic eggs available and use them in your recipes within a day or two.

Here's an example of a delicious dairy-free, soy-free smoothie that takes advantage of fresh summer fruit.

PEACHY CREAM SMOOTHIE

1 ripe fresh peach, skin removed (preferably organic)

1–2 scoops high-quality peach sorbet, naturally sweetened

¼ teaspoon vanilla extract

½ cup orange juice

3 tablespoons unsweetened coconut milk

1 fresh, high-quality, organic raw egg

dash sugar or Sucralose

With a paring knife (or your fingers if the peach is ripe enough), peel the skin off the peach and cut into chunks, taking care to avoid hard textures near the pit. Drop into a blender or tall glass with all other ingredients and blend to smooth consistency. If fresh, ripe peaches are out of season, use high-quality juice-packed canned peaches instead, and add a little of the juice to the smoothie for the consistency you like.

CASEIN-FREE EGGNOG FOR KIDS

This recipe lets everyone in on a great holiday tradition, and it is a fun novelty for kids who think eggnog only comes from supermarket cartons. The higher quality and fresher the egg, the better the nog. Pasteurized eggs do not perform as well in the recipe. Discard leftover nog after a day. This makes 8 half-cup servings. As a special holiday treat, soy milk is permissible in the recipe, but you can experiment with nut milks or other alternative milks. Increase the confectioner's sugar to 1/3 cup if you use unsweetened milks. Float some Hip Whip on top and sprinkle with nutmeg, freshly grated if you really want to make it pop.

4 fresh eggs
1/4 cup confectioner's sugar
2 cups Silk Soy Vanilla Creamer
2 cups almond milk
1/2 cup rice milk
1/4 teaspoon pumpkin pie spice
nutmeg

Separate the yolks from the whites. Beat the yolks well with the sugar until the mixture is smooth. Add 1 cup of the Silk Creamer, the other "milks," and pumpkin pie spice, and beat until thoroughly blended. Beat the whites separately with clean beaters, until soft peaks form. Fold these gently into the yolk mixture. Then slowly fold and stir in the remaining Silk Creamer. Pour out into serving cups with a spoonful of Hip Whip on top and sprinkle with nutmeg.

Wrapping It Up

Enjoy these new foods and recipes. There are hundreds more awaiting your perusal in books and on the Web. Using a special diet is well worth it when your child feels better, functions better, and grows better—which is, of course, what children deserve and need. Overcome any sense of separation this may create for you or your child by making enough for everybody, whenever reasonable. Most of the time, it disappears!

RESOURCES AND FURTHER READING

These days there are many excellent resources for families and providers endeavoring to understand children with learning and developmental disorders in a deeper context, rather than simply as children with troubled brain chemistry who need psychiatric medications. Treating the whole child works well, but it does challenge our health care system to rise to new heights, because it asks parents and providers to work as a team. It also means thinking holistically rather than in terms of body parts (brain, stomach, muscles, etc.), as doctors are trained to think. And it asks both parents and doctors to learn a lot, to sift through new information that may not have been covered in anybody's training. This does not mean the information is invalid. It means it is either new information, or a new way to apply old information.

Besides support with how to monitor your child's progress, provider resources, parent networking ideas, and suggested reading on related topics, this section offers resources for learning more about the science behind how the nutrition care described in this book works. Some of the items listed are peer-reviewed—that is, they have been scrutinized by the physician's professional peers and approved for publication in an academic journal. While some parents don't mind reading this stuff, it is heavy going, but it is usually what your doctor is looking for when he says he wants "proof" that using the tools described in this book are valid. You can either get the items mentioned here off the Internet (some are free, some are not) or give the academic references to your doctor, and let his staff obtain the articles if need be. There are hundreds of important academic research articles on the nutritional biochemistry and toxicity issues of autism—they are impossible to list here. Start with Bryan Jepson's book (see below), or the learning module I wrote (also below), if you need comprehensive bibliographies of peer review on the subject. There are also suggestions here for online parent support resources, so you can find providers, parents, or other tools to help you implement strategies that make your child learn, grow, and thrive.

READING ON THE BIOMEDICAL TREATMENT MODEL FOR AUTISM

Changing the Course of Autism: A Scientific Approach for Parents and Physicians, by Bryan Jepson, MD. Sentient Publications, 2007. This book gives a concise explanation of each layer that is treatable in children with autism spectrum disorders. It is suitable for both parents and providers because it is in language plain enough for parents to follow, but includes ample academic referencing for doctors to scrutinize if they like.

"Autism and Gastrointestinal Symptoms," review article, by Karoly Horvath, MD, PhD, and Jay A. Perman, MD. *Current Gastroenterology Reports* 2002, 4: 251–58. Current Science Inc. This is an academic article suitable for sharing with your pediatrician and gastroenterologist, if they are unfamiliar with the link between bowel symptoms, nutrition, and autism. It summarizes findings from several studies that describe the gastrointestinal problems found in children with autism spectrum disorders. If your doctor needs information about these issues in order to give effective care to your child, this is a good item to share or suggest.

"Medical Nutrition Therapy for Pediatric Autism: Strategies for Assessment and Monitoring," by Judy Converse, MPH, RD, LD. Continuing Education University, Ohio, 2008. I wrote this course module so health professionals could learn how to safely and effectively use special diets for autism in children. It includes over a hundred academic references to support why nutrition care matters for kids on the spectrum, so if your provider needs lots of proof, this would be a good way to share it. It is available as a PDF download at my own website, www.NutritionCare.net (print it out and put it in a three-ring binder; it is about 60 pages), or from Continuing Education University's website, www.CEU4U.com, as a course of study that awards credits to health professionals (with this option, licensed health professionals use the study module and testing tool via the Web). The academic references listed in this module cover methylation, oxidative stress, use of methylcobalamin, Opiate Theory, nutrition assessment tools, scientific review of the heavy metals issue, and more, so this is a one-stop-shopping item for doctors who need peer review on all these parts of the autism-diet story. It also includes diagnosis codes used by insurance companies for nutrition care, so providers can learn how to "code" their care in order to trigger payment for you.

"Dark Adaptation, Motor Skills, Docosahexaenoic Acid (DHA), and Dyslexia," by Jacqueline Stordy, PhD. *American Journal of Clinical Nutrition*, 2000, 71: 323–26, Supplement. This is one of the first academic articles to explain how the omega-3 fatty acid DHA supports learning, vision, and motor skills if replenished. There have been dozens of scientific articles published on the health benefits of omega-3 fatty acids. Dr. Stordy has also published a parent-friendly book on this important piece of the nutrition puzzle for kids with autism spectrum disorders, ADHD, sensory integration disorder, or learning, mood, and behavior problems: *The LCP Solution* (Random House, 2001). Another helpful book for parents on this topic is *The Omega 3 Connection*, by Andrew Stoll, MD (Free Press, 2001).

"Is Autism a G-Alpha Protein Defect Reversible with Natural Vitamin A?," by Mary Megson, MD, FAAP. *Medical Hypotheses* 2000, 54: 979–83S. I have highlighted this article because poor eye contact is such a hallmark of autism, and behavioral interventions for it are common. But Dr. Megson's work explains why, biochemically, making direct eye contact may only show a splintered visual field for persons with autism. Part of Dr. Megson's theory is that the mechanism that makes frontal vision possible can be damaged by DTaP vaccine. She elucidates how this mechanism may be repaired by replenishing a naturally occurring form of vitamin A called cis-palmitate, found in cod liver oil. In practice, I have repeatedly seen cod liver oil improve or even abruptly restore eye contact in children with autism, when given at ordinary doses. This article may help your providers understand one piece of the nutrition puzzle for a child with autism who refuses eye contact. If Dr. Megson's hypothesis is correct, children with autism who avoid eye contact may see quite poorly via frontal vision. Her presentation on how the eye functions in this circumstance is poignant. It reveals a broken visual field with fragments visible only on the periphery, and little visible in front. In this situation, a child with autism can't see you when you demand direct eye contact, but sees you better when looking to the side. Forcing eye contact by holding the child's chin would then not only be ineffective, but border on cruelty, because it makes the child strain through scattered visual fragments that don't make sense. This may heighten anxiety and avoidance behavior in many affected children, not improve it. If your child is unable to make eye contact, using cod liver oil is a safe place to start. Read Dr. Megson's article or share it with your provider if you like.

Children with Starving Brains: A Medical Treatment Guide for Autism Spectrum Disorder, by Jaquelyn McCandless, MD. Bramble Books, 2002. A helpful parent guide that explains what DAN doctors do, and how this might help children on the spectrum.

BOOKS ABOUT VACCINATION

Many parents feel confused and concerned about vaccination. These books may help. As you will be pressed to give your child booster shots again and again throughout elementary school, adolescence, college years, and even in the childbearing years, you will want to have every confidence that they are beneficial and not harmful in your child's case. Children now receive over ninety vaccinations by age eighteen, with most administered after two years of age. This degree of vaccination is unprecedented; it has never been done before, and there is no other medicine that we force unilaterally on everyone. Its role as a trigger for neurodevelopmental disorders, learning disabilities, juvenile diabetes, and allergies is still debated.

The books listed discuss the risks versus benefits of using the recommended vaccine schedule, as well as information you can use to make choices for your family. There are many other titles about vaccines once you enter this genre, but these represent some of the earliest and strongest out there. If you choose to defer any vaccines, learn about other health care tools such as good nutrition and naturopathic or homeopathic care. These create and support robust immunity in children, and can help you manage and treat illnesses when they occur. If you are interested in your state's laws regarding vaccine choice, visit www.NVIC.org and click on your state.

What Your FDoctor May Not Tell You About Children's Vaccinations, by
    Stephanie Cave, MD. Warner Books, 2001.
The Vaccine Guide: Risks and Benefits for Children and Adults, by Randall Neustaedter, OMD. North Atlantic Books, 2002.
What Every Parent Should Know About Childhood Immunization, by
    Jamie Murphy. Jamie Murphy, 1993 (10th printing, 2005).
When Your Doctor Is Wrong: Hepatitis B Vaccine & Autism, by Judy
    Converse, MPH, RD, LD. XLibris, 2002.
*Evidence of Harm. Mercury in Vaccines and the Autism Epidemic: A
    Medical Controversy*, by David Kirby. St. Martin's Press, 2005.
A Shot in the Dark, by Harris Coulter, PhD, and Barbara Loe Fisher.
    Avery Press, 1990.
Raising a Vaccine Free Child, by Wendy Lydall, 2005.

What about the MMR vaccine? This has stirred more controversy for families affected by autism than any other issue. Most pediatricians were satisfied that the shot was exonerated in recent years, in a large study that has become known as the Danish Study. But many fervently disagree still, based on these two items, which should be read by any interested pediatrician or parent:

"Commentary: MMR and Autism in Perspective—The Denmark Story," by Carol Stott, PhD, Mark Blaxill, and Andrew Wakefield, MB, FRCS. *Journal of American Physicians and Surgeons* 9, no. 3 (Fall 2004). Available online at www.whale.to/vaccine/stott.pdf. This review rebuts the Danish Study and disagrees with its conclusions. It illustrates how a causal link between MMR vaccine and autism is actually *supported* by the Danish Study data, and exposes a design flaw that concealed rising cases of autism in the data set.

"Pediatric Vaccines Influence Primate Behavior, and Amygdala Growth and Opioid Ligand Binding," by Laura Hewittson, University of Pittsburgh. This study is still in production at the time of this publication, but it deserves mention because it is the first of its kind, and it represents a well-coordinated effort among several scientists from universities around the country. It is essentially a safety review that many parents and pediatricians alike assume was completed long ago. It tested effects of giving vaccines in the same sequence that U.S. infants now receive them. This was done because vaccines are tested and licensed individually, but the safety of the vaccine schedule in total had never been reviewed. In all test animals (monkeys), "progressively severe, chronic, active inflammation" was found in GI tissue, along with changes in gene expression and "significant neurodevelopmental deficits" that were consistent with autism. This is a benchmark study that should be of keen interest to all pediatricians. Its findings shout out the need for review of vaccine policy and practice, and the timing and number of vaccines given to children today in particular.

RESOURCES FOR WELL CHILD CARE

Some families feel better using naturopathic, nutritional, or homeopathic measures for well child care, with pharmacological strategies used as infrequently as possible. You can have providers on your team who are trained to provide these helps safely and effectively. If your pediatrician lacks this expertise, consider switching to one who has it.

Naturopathic doctors, osteopaths, family practice physicians, or licensed family nurse practitioners can provide school physicals, order lab tests, monitor growth, and help your child through routine illnesses. Ideally, keep a medical provider in the loop who can make specialist referrals when needed, and who has admitting privileges at your area's pediatric hospital. If you have had a falling-out with your pediatrician, consider asking a family practice physician to help. A classically trained homeopath can be a great addition to your team, for helping your child push more quickly through illnesses, recover from injuries or surgeries, address behavior challenges, or to manage chronic conditions such as asthma, chronic fatigue, or learning or developmental diagnoses. While the scientific method has so far not been able to explain *how* homeopathy works, it has been used to show that it often does work, in many clinical trials. Like any tool, homeopathy is most effective when administered by an experienced provider, especially for chronic, entrenched conditions. We also don't know exactly how or why many medications work (aspirin, some psychiatric drugs), but we have seen that they do work. Check these sites for individuals in your locale who can help:

- www.Naturopathic.org, the American Association of Naturopathic Physicians
- www.Homeopathy-Cures.com/search.html, for a listing by state of classical homeopaths
- www.HomeopathyHome.com, for books, discussion groups, and resources
- www.abcHomeopathy.com, for an interactive "Remedy Finder" feature lets you identify which remedies best match your symptoms
- *Everybody's Guide to Homeopathic Medicines: Safe and Effective Remedies for You and Your Family*, by Stephen Cummings, MD, and Dana Ullman, MPH. North Atlantic Books, 2004. I have a dog-eared 1990s edition of this book in my home and

have relied on it to treat minor colds, stomach bugs, stings, scrapes, bangs, sleep problems, and more. But don't take my word for it—this book is praised by Dr. Andrew Weil himself.

■ www.SokHop.com (Save Our Kids, Heal Our Planet), an initiative to educate parents on how to raise healthy children in a toxic-overloaded world. Organic foods, good nutrition, eco-friendly initiatives, vaccine choice, autism/ADHD recovery, and well child care alternatives are the emphasis at their expos and conferences.

HELPFUL WEBSITES FOR FAMILIES AFFECTED BY AUTISM

By now, there are countless nonprofits serving those with autism. This makes it an easier path to walk than it was even a few years ago. Especially helpful are electronic mailing lists, blogs, and opportunities to connect online with other parents in similar situations. Many parents of children with autism rarely get vacations, time away as a couple, or time to socialize with other families. The Internet can fill some of this painful void. One of my favorite features is on the Generation Rescue website, which has a spot to click on a "Rescue Angel"—this is a parent in your area who has volunteered to offer moral support. Take advantage of these resources, and you will find you have a lot of company.

■ www.GenerationRescue.org, for information on hopeful treatments, and your local parent and provider resources
■ www.hriptc.org, for a booklet on metallothionein and autism
■ Talk About Curing Autism (TACA), for information, research, and referrals on recovery and treatment strategies for autism
■ www.Autism-Society.org (Autism Society of America), for education strategies, resources, and legislative updates for families affected by autism
■ www.Autism.com (Autism Research Institute), for resources for biomedical treatments, the Autism Evaluation Checklist, and more

- www.AutismSpeaks.org (Autism Speaks), for nationwide research news, volunteer opportunities, resources, and legislative updates. Founded in 2005 and now perhaps the largest of all autism nonprofits out there, Autism Speaks has begun to include initiatives other than genetics in its research funding.

MONITORING YOUR CHILD'S PROGRESS

You can use a tool called the Autism Treatment Evaluation Checklist, available at www.autism.com/ari/atec/atec-online.htm, to follow your child's progress with any intervention you are using. This was developed by the Autism Research Institute in San Diego and has been used by thousands of families, as well as in some research efforts. It is an impartial way to track how well your intervention is going. Check the Autism Research Institute's site (www.autism.com) for other tools, resources, and referrals for parents as well.

CALORIE RECOMMENDATIONS FOR CHILDREN

The Food and Nutrition Board of the Institute of Medicine (National Institutes of Health) published these recommendations in 2005, for total energy intakes in children (that is, total calorie intakes), based on years of review with several data sources. You can use these to judge whether or not your child's total food intake is too low or too high. Add up your child's calories for a day or two, and see if they are in the right range. These are suggestions for typically growing and developing children. Calorie needs go up in underweight or growth-delayed children, with chronic illness, and with physical trauma. For babies, calorie needs also rise with chronic crying, screaming syndrome,* or chronic sleeplessness.

---

* Screaming syndrome is a feature of an adverse vaccine reaction that causes infants to scream violently and incessantly for several hours. The baby's back may arch rigidly and limbs may tremor; he cannot be soothed, take feedings, or fall asleep. The baby becomes breathless, red-faced, or even blue with effort. Babies with screaming syndrome should go to an emergency room for evaluation.

The calories needed are shown per pound as well as per kilogram here, because parents usually think in pounds in the United States, while other countries use kilograms and so does the Food and Nutrition Board.

AGE	CALORIES PER POUND PER DAY	CALORIES PER KILOGRAM PER DAY
0–6 months	37–49	82–107
6–12 months	37	82
1–3 years	46	102
4–6 years	41	90
7–10 years	32	70
11–14 years	25 (boys), 21 (girls)	55 (boys), 47 (girls)

HOW TO DETERMINE YOUR CHILD'S IDEAL BODY WEIGHT

For kids, being too skinny can be unhealthy and dangerous, just as being too fat can be unhealthy and dangerous. As explained in Chapter 2, simply plotting your child's weight for age is not enough information to tell whether or not a child's weight is healthy. This is because by the time weight begins to slip, a child has already been in a nutrition deficit for a while. When height begins to slip, too, this means that a nutrition problem has been there even longer; intervention is definitely appropriate. Most children I meet who tumble down their growth charts have not been referred for nutrition assessment (their parents call me on their own), because pediatricians often do not notice a nutrition problem until it is so far entrenched, the child has been struggling for a long time. Usually by this time, specialists who can't fix the problem have been called in, to no avail (neurologists, psychologists, allergists, psychiatrists, behavior therapists, and so on). Even children who flounder for years below the 5th percentile for weight to height ratio may get no referral for nutrition care. The reason is that pediatricians frequently skip review of this parameter, and mistakenly think all is well enough. Culturally, we often think being really skinny is okay for kids, and that the only problem is being too fat. But being too thin for age and height can trigger many problems for children, in terms of learning, immune function, and development.

Weight to height ratio and ideal body weight (IBW) are two growth parameters that can tell you if your child is just skinny but healthy, or dangerously thin for his height. Being too thin means your child can get sick more often, can get more complications with illness, and will have a harder time with school tasks, socializing, behavior, or attention and focus. It may also mean that developmental milestones such as potty training, talking appropriately, or self-feeding and self-care skills will be more elusive. So it is important to know the difference between just being a skinny kid, and being dangerously underweight or growth-compromised.

Besides the usual charts that follow your child's weight and height for age—the ones you may have seen in the pediatrician's office—the CDC makes growth charts that show the weight to height ratio for your child. This chart is called the weight for stature chart. It relates a child's weight to his height, to tell you if it is proportionate and healthy. You can download a weight for stature chart from the CDC's website (www.CDC.gov) by putting "growth charts" in their search engine. Scroll down this page to the bottom, and pick from the choices for "Optional Charts" for your child's age and sex. Once you click on the chart you want, it loads onto your computer screen and you can print it out. It is obvious how to use it; simply plot the point where your child's weight on one axis meets his height on the other. Weight for stature charts are usually used for infants and young children. After about age four or five, clinicians switch to the body mass index (BMI) charts, which is another way to screen whether your child is at a good weight for his height. BMI is a growth parameter that can be used for adults, too. It is useful for checking whether children are becoming overweight or obese, and may be less sensitive for catching children who are approaching underweight status. On either chart, children should follow a steady pattern. Dropping down more than 20 points to a lower percentile can mean that a child is stuck in a total calorie deficit, or has had a chronic illness, a significant physical trauma, or something that triggered malabsorption of his or her diet. Occasionally, it can mean that a really chubby baby has simply become a leaner toddler. This is fine, as long as the weight to height ratio is not slipping below the 10th percentile, the child's height is not slowing down, and the child is otherwise entirely well and typical.

Ideal body weight (IBW) is another way to check whether your child is in the too-thin category. A child's IBW is the 50th percentile weight for the child's current height—that is, it's the weight that is the most typical and healthy for any particular height. Your child should weigh at least 90 percent of his IBW; below this, he is in malnutrition and will suffer the effects of that. For example, if a child's IBW is 50 pounds, then he must weigh at least 90 percent of 50 pounds (which is 45 pounds) to be in healthy nutrition status. If he weighs less than 45 pounds, then malnutrition is present and creating its own problems for cognition, behavior, and so on.

To find the ideal body weight for your child, you need your child's height, her actual weight now (don't guess; weigh her without a diaper or with minimal clothing), and a weight for stature chart.* Once you know your child's weight, then measure your child's height accurately. No shoes or socks, heels against the wall, legs and spine straight, and have your child stand with hips/buttocks, shoulders, and head touching the wall. Mark the wall by laying a pencil horizontally on the crown of your child's head and letting the pencil point touch the wall. Once you've got the mark, you can measure it later; no need for your child to wait stock still while you fiddle with a yardstick or tape measure. For infants or toddlers who are not able to stand this way for you, have them lie flat and straight, and mark the floor in the

*This works for children 30–48 inches tall. Smaller, younger children can use the weight for length chart instead, and older children can use body mass index for age charts to check whether they are truly underweight.

same way. You can also use art roll paper and lay your child on this, so you can mark it. Measure it after you've got the marks you need.

Next, use the weight for stature chart to locate the 50th percentile weight for this height. Find the point where your child's actual height meets the 50th percentile point for weight. This is your child's ideal body weight. If he is above this by a little, that is okay. If you're not sure whether your child is too heavy, use the body mass index chart; above the 85th percentile BMI for age means your child is probably too heavy. If your child weighs less than the ideal body weight you found, then you can check if he is *too* far below it with this equation:

$$\frac{\text{Your child's current actual weight}}{\text{50th percentile weight for height}} \times 100 = \%IBW$$

The percent ideal body weight (%IBW) should be at least 90. Here's an example: A five-year-old boy is 45 inches tall and weighs 40 pounds. On the height for age chart, that places him at the 90th percentile. On the weight for age chart, he lands just under the 50th percentile. His pediatrician thinks this looks fine. Next, we can use the boys' weight for stature chart. Find the boy's height, 45 inches, on the stature (horizontal) axis. Then place a ruler on that point and align it vertically, to locate weight at the 50th percentile. It is 44.5 pounds. This is the ideal body weight for a boy who is five years old and 45 inches tall. He only weighs 40 pounds. Let's check if this is too thin.

$$\frac{\text{40 pounds current actual weight}}{\text{44.5 ideal body weight}} \times 100 = 89.8\%$$

This means he is in mild malnutrition, and too thin for his height. He needs to gain weight to function better, but the pediatrician doesn't know this just by plotting weight for age and height for age. Being near 90 percent of ideal body weight for a child is not great, so this is not hairsplitting. Once a child drops below that level, based on large data sets reviewed over the decades, it means that infection fighting, cognition, and other functions are compromised.

NUTRITION DIAGNOSIS CODES

When nutrition care is the correct measure for a child, insurance should pay for it, but your billing statements will need the correct codes to help that happen. A common error made by biomedical providers is using diagnosis codes for what are considered purely psychiatric or developmental disorders on billing statements that describe nutrition problems. This will be reliably rejected by health insurers— who, in their Byzantine nonlogic—persist in the view that autism is a purely psychiatric or neurological disorder that warrants only brain scans and medications for care. While your insurer may pay for an MRI of your child's brain without flinching if the diagnosis code is autism ($1500–$3500), it may buck you to the grave if you'd like three visits of appropriate nutrition care (about $500). Three is usually the number of visits a child in my care needs to get under way and start getting better, which is a lot more than a brain scan can do. Billing statements for nutrition care or biomedical treatments should describe the problems they are treating, not autism. Below is a list of some helpful codes. You can print this out from www.NutritionCare .net and share it with your providers or health insurer to find out how coverage may apply for these conditions.

789.0 abdominal pain	278.0 obesity/other hyperalimentation
536.9 gastric retention	278.01 morbid obesity
536.8 acid peptic disease	783.6 hyperalimentation NOS
535.40 allergic gastritis	787.91 diarrhea
558.3 allergic diarrhea	V15.02 allergy to milk products
558.9 allergic colitis	V15.03 allergy to eggs

995.3 allergy unspecified

283.9 anemia

783.0 anorexia

493.9 asthma

314.01 ADD

789.0 colic

564.0 constipation

782.1 dermatitis, unspecified

250.0 diabetes mellitus

054.0 eczema herpeticum

287.0 allergic purpura

693.1 dermatitis, foods

629.9 eczema

783.4 failure to thrive, NOS

783.41 failure to thrive, child

783.42 delayed milestones

783.3 feeding problems, infant/elder

783.43 short stature

783.5 polydipsia

783.6 polyphagia

783.7 FTT adult

774.6 hyperbilirubinemia

783.1 abnormal weight gain

783.2 abnormal weight loss

783.22 underweight

V30.2 newborn care

780.3 seizure disorder

520.7 teething

263.1 mild malnutrition

265.2 pallegra

266.2 other B complex deficiency

268.0 rickets, active

963.5 poisoning by vitamin preparations

253.8 adiposigenital dystrophy

259.9 obesity endocrine origin NOS

278.1 localized adiposity

270.9 amino acid metabolic disorder NOS

250.9 diabetes mellitus

272.2 mixed hyperlipidemia

272.4 other-NOS hyperlipidemia

271.3 disaccharidease insufficiency

271.3 lactose malabsorption

280.1 iron deficiency due to poor intake

281.0 pernicious anemia

280.9 iron deficiency NOS

268.9 vit D def

275.9 mineral metab disorder NOS

275.1 disorders copper metabolism

579.8 food intolerance

558.9 gastroenteritis

564.1 irritable bowel syndrome

278.2 hypervitaminosis A

307.42 insomnia

277.1 disorders of porphyrin metabolism

277.2 disorders purine/pyrimidine metabolism

277.9 unspecified disorder metabolism

112.85 candidal enteritis

251.2 hypoglycemia unspecified

261 nutritional marasmus

263.0 moderate calorie malnutrition

265.0 beriberi

266.1 pyridoxine deficiency

267 vitamin C deficiency

268.2 osteomalacia, unspecified

269.2 vitamin deficiency NOS   269.3 mineral deficiency NOS

269.9 nutritional deficiency NOS   277.99 cystic fibrosis

579.1 tropical sprue   269.9 underweight/debility

579.0 gluten induced enteropathy   577.8 pancreatic insufficiency

529.0 glossitis

A number of diagnosis codes describe intestinal infections. Some types of microbial overgrowth that I have observed on stool cultures of children in my caseload are described here with codes. There are many more than these. Providers can use these codes to justify treatment measures with antimicrobial herbs or drugs, or to justify consultation on specific probiotics.

008.3	proteus mirabilis
008.4	other specified bacteria
008.41	staphylococcus
008.42	pseudomonas
008.43	campylobacter
008.46	other anaerobic bacteria
008.47	other gram negative bacteria
008.49	other organisms
008.5	bacterial enteritis unspecified
008.6	enteritis to specified virus

LAB TESTS QUICK REFERENCE GUIDE

This is a fast-glance chart for the tests described in more detail in Chapter 3.

Biochemistry Studies and Medical Procedures Common
for Autism Spectrum Disorders

TEST	PURPOSE: TO RULE OUT OR DETERMINE
CBC with differential	Anemias, red or white blood cell abnormalities
Endoscopy, gut biopsy	GI disease, gut inflammation, ulcers, reflux damage, pancreatic function, nodularity
MRI and SPECT scan	Structural brain abnormalities, hypoperfused regions
IgE/RAST	Food allergy/anaphylaxis
IgG/ELISA	Food sensitivity/delayed inflammatory response
Tissue transglutaminase antibody, reticulin antibody, endomysial antibody	Antibodies specific to celiac disease
Antigliadin IgG, IgA	Antibodies specific to gluten sensitivity
Urine toxic metals*	Excretion of heavy metals (measured after provoking agent)
Stool toxic metals	Excretion of heavy metals (measured after provoking agent)
Urea cycle disorders screening	Inherited disorders of urea cycle
Urine metabolic organic acids	Functional vitamin and mineral status
Urine microbial organic acids	Acids produced by disruptive gut flora
Urine polypeptides	Dietary protein absorbed as opiate-like peptides
Urine pyrroles	Kryptopyrroluria (functional zinc or B6 deficit)
Urine porphyrins	Indirect measure of heavy metal toxicity
Serum fatty acids, triene to tetraene ratio	Essential fatty acid status
Liver function testing	Liver stress from diet, drugs, inherited disorders
Genetic screening	Inherited syndromes
Serum amino acids	Mitochondrial or inherited disorders of metabolism
Urine amino acids	Inherited disorders of metabolism
Muscle biopsy	Mitochondrial disorder
Digestive stool analysis	Indirect screen for maldigestion, gut inflammation, flora, parasites; includes stool culture and sensitivity
Stool microbiology analysis	Stool culture and sensitivity for yeast, parasites, and bacteria

TEST	PURPOSE: TO RULE OUT OR DETERMINE
Thyroid studies	Thyroid function
Total Cholesterol, HDL, LDL	Cholesterol screening
Anti-Streptolysin-O (ASO) titer	Antibodies to streptococcal bacteria
Serum lactulose and mannitol	Intestinal permeability marker
Serum lactate, glutathione, ammonia	Oxidative stress markers
Ceruloplasmin, serum copper, copper to zinc ratio	Unbound copper screen, zinc status
Plasma cysteine, methionine	Methylation capacity

*Blood is not valid for heavy metals screening because blood only informs on active or recent exposures. Past exposures presumably sequestered in fatty tissue must be "provoked" with an agent like Chemet to be measured. Excreted metals are then measured in stool/urine collection.

INDEX

Page numbers in **bold** indicate tables; page numbers followed by "n" indicate notes.